"This book is a most in-depth and user-friendly approach to a serious and, in some cases, debilitating disease. The authors speak with great experience and, as a result, have produced a work that any Sjögren's syndrome patient, family member, and/or health professional should have to help navigate the course of treatment for this fascinating yet mysterious disease."

> —Stuart S. Kassan, MD, FACP, Past Chair of the SSF Medical and Scientific Advisory Board, and Clinical Professor of Medicine, University of Colorado Health Sciences Center, Denver

"As a Sjögren's Syndrome researcher and clinician I heartily applaud your efforts and believe strongly that a person is his or her own best advocate for health and that education is the key to managing a chronic disease like Sjögren's Syndrome."

> —Janine A. Smith, MD, Deputy Clinical Director, National Eye Institute, National Institutes of Health

"A thoughtful and moving guide to surviving not only Sjögren's Syndrome but also to living with any chronic vulnerability. Helps all those of us perplexed by an awareness of mortality that the authors so courageously and rationally face."

> —Harold J. Bursztajn, MD, senior Harvard Medical School faculty physician, and practitioner of psychoanalytically informed psychiatry in Cambridge, Massachusetts

"The authors of the *Survival Guide* urge us to live authentically, and they have given us their hard-won but gentle wisdom for doing so. They shine a light into our doctors' offices, our relationships, and our innermost fears, and they teach us that we can live and live well with Sjögren's syndrome. Bravo!"

> —Susan Milstrey Wells, author, *A Delicate Balance: Living Successfully with Chronic Illness*

"This book offers the reader a thorough and accurate understanding of Sjögren's Syndrome and provides real-life scenarios of what it is like to live with this disorder. It should be helpful to patients, their families and friends, and the doctors who treat them."

> —Carol Esposito, Psy.D., psychologist, Sjögren's Patient

The Sjögren's Syndrome
SURVIVAL GUIDE

Teri P. Rumpf, Ph.D.

Katherine Morland Hammitt

New Harbinger Publications, Inc.

Publisher's Note

This publication is designed to provide accurate and authoritative information in regard to the subject matter covered. It is sold with the understanding that the publisher is not engaged in rendering psychological, financial, legal, or other professional services. If expert assistance or counseling is needed, the services of a competent professional should be sought.

Distributed in the U.S.A. by Publishers Group West; in Canada by Raincoast Books; in Great Britain by Hi Marketing, Ltd.; in South Africa by Real Books, Ltd.; in Australia by Boobook; and in New Zealand by Tandem Press.

Copyright © 2003 by Teri P. Rumpf, and Katherine Morland Hammitt
New Harbinger Publications, Inc.
5674 Shattuck Avenue
Oakland, CA 94609

Cover design by Lightbourne Images
Text design by Tracy Marie Carlson

ISBN 1-57224-356-2 Paperback

New Harbinger Publications' Web site address: www.newharbinger.com

05   04   03

10   9   8   7   6   5   4   3   2   1

First printing

To Noah

and

To Kelsey, Kenneth, Harry, and Kathy's parents

Who helped us see life as a celebration and supported us through the tough times.

Contents

Foreword

One of the greatest gifts patients with a chronic illness like Sjögren's syndrome can receive is knowledge—not only about the disease itself but about ways to help themselves. Through years of clinical and research experience with Sjögren's syndrome patients, we have discovered that people who take an active role in their own care reap benefits that help them cope better with day-to-day living and the inevitable ups and downs of dealing with a chronic illness. In Sjögren's syndrome, medicine does not offer easy answers or solutions, making patient involvement and a willingness to learn that much more essential.

Many patients who come to our Sjögren's syndrome medical clinics are very concerned when they are first diagnosed. Usually, they have never heard of Sjögren's syndrome. We, as physicians, are here to help, as are our dental, nursing, and other professional colleagues. The Sjögren's Syndrome Foundation is an excellent resource for information and support, as are books such as this one. Today, there is also considerable information available relevant to Sjögren's syndrome through the Internet from foundations, universities, and government, including the National Institutes of Health. This information can empower patients to make a difference in their own lives.

How? By learning about Sjögren's syndrome and its symptoms and by understanding that each person's experience with this disease is unique. Patients can reduce their anxiety and help their doctors take better care of them as well. They need to know their symptoms are real and not just "in their head." As awareness of Sjögren's syndrome increases, physicians are now better able to treat many of its major manifestations. However, some problems such as fatigue and the psychological impact of this disease may still be underrecognized and go untreated.

Seeking opportunities to learn about other patients' day-to-day experience with Sjögren's syndrome can help patients understand their own. This book offers readers a chance to focus on the biological, social, and psychological aspects of living with a chronic illness, as well as enhancing their ability to cope and in some ways to heal.

The Sjögren's Syndrome Survival Guide offers a wealth of knowledge about Sjögren's in an easy-to-understand format. It is also an excellent resource for patients' families, friends, and health care providers, because it communicates the difficulty of living with this disease and the important role of support. By reading this book and taking an active part in the management of their disease, patients will be well on the way to acquiring the knowledge and skills to develop one of the most powerful tools of all—the power to help themselves. For many, these tools can represent the first steps toward taking back control of their lives.

Patients should become true partners with their doctors. This book can be viewed as a helpful companion to *The New Sjögren's Syndrome Foundation Handbook* (see Resources); these two books provide different kinds of information about Sjögren's syndrome and, together, can help patients achieve this goal.

Katherine Hammitt, a Sjögren's patient and journalist, has long worked with the Sjögren's Syndrome Foundation to ensure better lives and hope for the future for those with Sjögren's. She helps readers understand this disease, what is known, and, just as important, what is not known. She has heard the many questions patients have had without receiving clear answers.

Teri Rumpf, a clinical psychologist and author as well as a Sjögren's patient, addresses psychological aspects, from dealing with the roller coaster of emotions that come with a chronic illness to the impact on relationships and work. Many patients will recognize themselves in the stories illustrating the day-to-day struggles of living with Sjögren's and find tips on how to cope more fruitfully with those struggles.

All patients and those who care about them will find *The Sjögren's Syndrome Survival Guide* to be invaluable. This book reminds all of us that people with Sjögren's syndrome are not alone in their journey to find better physical and emotional health. By addressing two important needs—medical information and the psychosocial aspects of illness—the authors have created a truly unique resource that will not only assist patients and families to better understand and cope with this devastating disorder but also, hopefully, enable them to lead healthier and more productive lives.

—Stanley R. Pillemer, MD
Sjögren's Syndrome Clinic
National Institutes of Dental and Craniofacial Research
National Institutes of Health

—Frederick B. Vivino, MD, FACR
Director, University of Pennsylvania Sjögren's Syndrome Center
Chief of Rheumatology, Presbyterian Medical Center University
of Pennsylvania Health System Philadelphia

Preface

In real life, illness isn't like it is in the movies. This is especially true when the disease is Sjögren's syndrome, and few people know what it is or have ever heard of it. In films, illness seems to enhance character. People are always there to help, the hero or heroine comes to some sort of illuminated understanding about life, and there are never any long waits for a doctor's appointment or problems with insurance companies. In the movie version, illness brings people and families together. Old quarrels are healed, ailing relationships are restored, and enemies make peace. Everyone looks good, even when they are very sick. On-screen, money is never an issue and the crisis comes out all right in the end. If the protagonist should eventually die, he or she is a better person by the time that happens, usually quite near the end of the film.

Life rarely follows art. In real life, a chronic illness like Sjögren's syndrome, or any of the diseases which occur concurrently with Sjögren's (lupus, rheumatoid arthritis, fibromyalgia, and scleroderma among them), may take years to diagnose, and patients are often misdiagnosed and misguided along the way. For some, the presence of disease is not acknowledged until vague and seemingly unrelated signs and symptoms eventually form a pattern that can be recognized and diagnosed. It is not uncommon for people with Sjögren's to have it for years before this happens. They wonder what is going on and why they really feel the way they do. All too frequently, they are told that the symptoms are all in their heads, or that no physical cause can be found. The lack of answers is frustrating and frightening.

Autoimmune diseases, the category of diseases to which Sjögren's syndrome belongs, are difficult to diagnose and treat. Part of the reason is that the symptoms can be vague and disparate; they occur in parts of the body that seem unrelated. Another reason is that symptoms remit and relapse; they come and go, and may or may not show up on laboratory analysis. Yet another reason is that physicians do not consider Sjögren's when making the diagnosis. Many still consider it a disease of dry eyes and dry mouth, not a systemic disease. Many do not think about it at all.

Even once a diagnosis has been established, the words "Sjögren's syndrome" do not evoke great concern or sympathy. Hardly anyone ever says, "Oh no, you have Sjögren's! You must do everything you can to take care of yourself! You must rest when you need to, you must not push yourself too hard!" Instead, it is our feeling that the majority of patients make extraordinary efforts to carry on, despite their symptoms, and frequently do more than their bodies willingly allow. The lack of understanding and information about Sjögren's makes people feel isolated.

This book is a guide for patients, physicians, families, and friends. Both authors have Sjögren's syndrome. We hope to make this the book that wasn't available to us years ago, when we were first diagnosed. Neither of us knows the moment when her illness first began. Between us, we have a great deal of experience with what Sjögren's can do.

We differentiate between "illness" and "disease," a distinction made by Dr. Arthur Kleinman in his book *The Illness Narratives* (1988). By *illness*, we mean all of the symptoms as they are perceived by the person who experiences them. Illness is the way an individual responds to his or her symptoms, the way he or she lives with them from day to day. When we say *disease*, we use the term to describe the signs of the disorder and, in effect, what a physician sees. Disease is a more objective state; it is illness from the outside.

We also use another word, *syndrome*. A syndrome is a set of signs that form a recognizable pattern and remain constant over time. New signs and symptoms emerge, while others remit, but all are consistent with the pattern or patterns of the syndrome. We use the word *chronic* to indicate a disease which may relapse and remit, but which, by definition, never goes away. Even if not active, it remains present, a lurker in the body, ready to make itself known at some future time.

It is easy to commit these words to paper, but difficult to live with this illness called Sjögren's syndrome. The presence of a chronic illness changes things. It affects the way we live our lives, relate to others, make plans, and set goals. This book is not only about what Sjögren's is, but also about how to live with it. Sjögren's is a disease that can vary widely in scope and intensity. It can remain mild or be debilitating. A chronic disease is unpredictable, and, in turn, having one makes life less predictable.

Over time, patterns emerge. If our bodies are unpredictable, we become familiar with their unpredictability. We learn what helps and what hurts, and become experts at knowing our bodies. Some things we do make us feel better; other things make us worse. Experience is a powerful teacher, but not everything needs to be experienced directly. We hope that the following chapters will provide a wide range of useful information and will allow the reader to draw on both the research we have done and the experience of all who have contributed to this book. In addition, we hope these pages will enable each person who reads them to know that she or he is not alone.

Acknowledgments

Portions of this manuscript were read and edited by many different people, and we would like to take this opportunity to offer our sincere appreciation. We would like to thank: Carol Esposito, Psy.D.; Philip C. Fox, DDS; David Giansiracusa, MD; Bonnie Litton, MA; Joan Manny, RN; Harvey Mazer, MD; Bobette Morgan; J. Daniel Nelson, MD; Stanley Pillemer, MD; and Mala Rafik, JD. We are also indebted to Lady Felicity Tompkins of New Zealand and Rose Anne Leakan, RN, of NIH, for assistance with information, and to Martha Gillispie Robinson for her special support.

Jeffrey W. Wilson, MD, offered tremendous support throughout this project as well as thorough review and comments on medical chapters.

We also wish to thank the Sjögren's Syndrome Foundation for its support during our odyssey in assembling a book that has long been needed for patients; in particular, we want to thank Elaine Alexander, MD, Ph.D.; Evelyn Bromet, Ph.D.; Rhoda Dennison; Arthur Grayzel, MD; Stuart S. Kassan, MD; Ann Race; and Board Medical and Scientific Advisory Board members already listed above.

Spencer Smith of New Harbinger Publications helped at virtually every stage, and we thank him for his efforts to bring this book to publication.

Finally, we offer a special thanks to David Markun, without whose patience, friendship, and remarkable technical expertise this book would not have been possible.

Many other people helped in the creation of this book by offering their personal experiences. We appreciate the stories they have shared with us, although we have not named them for reasons of privacy. In the event we have omitted anyone, we regret that it was due to a temporary lapse; you have not been forgotten. To all, we thank you. For us, this has been a labor of love.

1

Sjögren's Syndrome: What Is That?

What is Sjögren's syndrome—a disease with a name that's so difficult to spell and pronounce? Sjögren's (SHOW-grins) syndrome is an autoimmune disease, a disease in which your body turns against itself, mistaking your own tissues for foreign invaders. Surprisingly, there are more than eighty autoimmune diseases, many of them overlapping, and Sjögren's is one of the most common. The Sjögren's Syndrome Foundation estimates that as many as four million Americans have Sjögren's syndrome, making it more common than better-known autoimmune diseases such as multiple sclerosis and lupus. It strikes women nine times more frequently than men and often takes more than six years for a diagnosis after symptoms start you on the search for answers from medical professionals (Boston Healthcare Associates 1996).

Any part of your body can be affected in Sjögren's syndrome, and patients will differ in the way they are affected by the disease, its severity, and the symptoms that are hardest to live with. Major targets of the autoimmune process in Sjögren's are the exocrine, or moisture-producing glands, resulting in the classic dry eyes and dry mouth. Most medical professionals identify these specific symptoms with Sjögren's, which complicates diagnosis when dry eyes and dry mouth are not there from the start or are not identified. Dry eyes and dry mouth, as we will explain later, can be more problematic than you might think, and dryness can have repercussions for many parts of the body, including the skin, vagina, gastrointestinal tract, and lungs. In addition to dryness, any body organ or system can be attacked by Sjögren's, sharing with other diseases a wide array of possible symptoms from joint and muscle pain to numbness and disabling fatigue, making it very difficult to carry on your normal, productive life.

To complicate matters, everyone with Sjögren's syndrome does not necessarily have the same symptoms or severity of disease. You might suffer from a mild case of dry eyes or dry mouth, while another person might have devastating dryness causing severe problems with seeing, eating, or talking, and yet someone else might have major organ involvement. We are not all alike. Our differences complicate diagnosis and often make it harder for physicians to know or explain to patients what might happen to them.

Sjögren's syndrome is chronic, meaning it lasts a lifetime. Right now, there is no cure, and more theories than answers abound about its cause. Treatments have been largely palliative, which means they can help you manage symptoms and feel better, but they don't help or stop the underlying problems. The future for treatment of Sjögren's, however, offers promise. Possibilities appearing in this new century of medicine are astonishing and accelerating every day. Researchers are pursuing new avenues, and a number of drugs have come on the market recently to help treat this disease. We also believe that you can have a tremendous impact on your illness by taking an active role in helping yourself. Understanding your illness and taking care of yourself are important for all patients, and especially the Sjögren's patient, in order to prevent or lessen serious complications and claim a better quality of life.

Definitions Can Change

How a disease is defined depends on what is known about that disease. As more is learned through research and experience, definitions and prognoses can change. A quick look at the evolving history of Sjögren's syndrome tells a great deal about how the disease is recognized and treated today. Sjögren's syndrome was named for

Dr. Henrik Sjögren, a Swedish doctor who found that some of his rheumatoid arthritis patients had dry mouth and dry eyes along with their joint pain. It was termed a "syndrome," which means a group of symptoms that occur together, and this term has remained. However, as we learn more about Sjögren's, we have found that Sjögren's is not just a description for a group of symptoms, but a separate and definable disease.

For a long time, Sjögren's syndrome was classified as a rheumatic, connective tissue disease, meaning that it affects the connective tissue, causing muscle and joint pain. Rheumatoid arthritis is a well-known example of a rheumatic disease and is one of several diseases that can accompany Sjögren's. Because of the involvement of connective tissue, Sjögren's can be classified as a form of arthritis. This is still true, but our perspective has broadened as we have come to understand how the symptoms occur: through an autoimmune process. Sjögren's is now most properly defined as an autoimmune disease.

Multiple Diagnoses

Sjögren's syndrome is a prime example of the crossover that can exist among autoimmune diseases. Approximately half of those with Sjögren's are diagnosed with another, major autoimmune disease. Complications that might accompany Sjögren's, such as autoimmune thyroid disorders or Raynaud's phenomenon (which causes vascular spasms), can also occur by themselves. The eighty-plus autoimmune diseases often overlap and you, unhappily, can have more than one. If your doctor diagnoses you with three different autoimmune diseases, this does not mean that two of the diagnoses are wrong, it means that you suffer from autoimmune disease, and your disease encompasses several overlapping or similar disorders, each with its own label.

Signs and Symptoms of Sjögren's

Because Sjögren's syndrome can affect any body organ or system, you can often have a disconcerting array of symptoms. It sometimes takes a physician or a patient who is a true detective to solve the puzzle. Rheumatologist Jeffrey Wilson calls the practice of medicine an art (Wilson 2001). Identifying and treating Sjögren's syndrome might call for more art than science.

Dry Eyes and Dry Mouth

The classic Sjögren's syndrome patient often presents with dry eyes or dry mouth. This means that the first symptom noticeable to either patient or doctor which leads to a diagnosis of Sjögren's will probably be dry eyes or dry mouth. When dryness is mild, the difficult first step is recognizing and identifying that your eyes or mouth are dry. For example, many people with mild dry mouth do not acknowledge that their mouth feels dry when asked. Instead, they just know they get a large number of cavities, no matter how many times they brush their teeth, or they drink a lot of liquid with food, or they begin finding that a glass of water next to their bed is necessary at night. One patient we know with Sjögren's, Ida, is fond of saying, "When it's the only mouth you've ever had, and you live with it all the time, you assume the way it feels is normal."

You might know your eyes burn and itch and are subject to frequent infections, but you might not know to call your eyes "dry." Other signs of dry eyes that might not be easily identified include feeling that sand or a foreign body is in your eyes or that light bothers you. Understanding dryness can be similar to recognizing blurred vision. Before those of us who need eyeglasses tried them for the first time, we probably would not have been able to describe our vision as blurry. Most of us just thought that the way we saw the world was the way everyone else saw it, and that no one could see the fine definition of the leaves on trees!

Of course, if you suffer from *severe* dryness, you'll know it! Your eyelids might stick to your eyeballs in the morning, or you might have difficulty swallowing or speaking. Your eyes and mouth might be very painful, and untreated dry eyes can lead to painful corneal abrasions and ulcers, at which point you'll surely get them checked. Dry mouth can cause painful oral ulcerations and yeast infections. Sadly, some Sjögren's patients are not diagnosed until their eyesight has become impaired or they have lost most of their teeth.

Dryness can have many causes, and Sjögren's syndrome is just one of them. Millions of people suffer from dry eyes or dry mouth, and not all of them or even most of them have Sjögren's. However, it's important to find out the cause. If you or your doctor is unaware of Sjögren's, you might not obtain a correct diagnosis or receive the correct treatment, or you might not be on the lookout for other complications that could occur elsewhere in your body. If you have Sjögren's syndrome, it's essential to have a correct diagnosis, so major complications can be prevented.

Dry Eyes: Possible Symptoms

* redness and irritation

* gritty feeling, as if you have sand or another foreign body in your eyes

* sensitivity to light (a condition called photophobia)

* pain

* sharp eye pain upon waking

* blurred vision that eyeglasses cannot correct

* increased symptoms after infrequent blinking, for example, after using the computer, watching television, or reading for long periods

* decreased tears

* recurring eye infections

* mucus

* crustiness, bumps, or redness around the eyelids (a condition called blepharitis, which can accompany dry eye)

* eyelids that do not move smoothly over the eye or that seem stuck to one's eyeballs, especially upon waking

Dry Mouth: Possible Symptoms

* rampant cavities

* cavities in unusual places, such as along the gum line, under fillings, and along cutting edges of teeth

- teeth erosion, chipping, and cracking
- difficulty chewing and swallowing food
- feeling as if you are choking when trying to swallow food
- dry, sticky surfaces on the inside of your mouth
- food sticking easily to the teeth
- difficulty speaking
- frequent need to drink liquids, especially when eating or speaking
- mouth sores or ulcers
- oral infections (while yeast or thrush infection usually appears white and patchy, in dry mouth these infections are sometimes bright red)
- burning, irritated mouth
- red, dry, furrowed tongue
- difficulty with dentures, especially with proper fitting
- bad breath
- cracking at the corners of your mouth
- loss of taste, or frequent metallic taste
- hoarseness
- dry cough
- persistent sore throat

Dryness Anywhere and Everywhere

Moisture-producing glands are everywhere in your body, so dryness can be felt in many ways. Nasal and sinus passages can be affected, becoming clogged with mucus and making you prone to infection. Many people with Sjögren's suffer frequent and prolonged sinus infections. Your dry throat can hurt and cause a constant cough. Ears and skin might itch. Sexual intercourse can be painful for women with Sjögren's because of decreased vaginal secretions, and they can be prone to vaginal infections. If the lining of the lungs is dry, pulmonary function can be affected, and infections, such as recurring bronchitis or pneumonia, can become a problem. Lack of saliva affects digestion, as does the reduced pancreatic enzyme production that can accompany Sjögren's. Lack of moisture in the gastrointestinal tract may cause constipation or an irritable bowel resulting in diarrhea. You may have difficulty eating highly spiced or acidic foods because they can burn the inside of your mouth or make sensitive digestion worse. Reflux is also a common problem.

Other Complications of Dryness

* itchy or flaky skin

* itchy ears

* nasal congestion and stuffiness

* frequent nose bleeds

* diminished sense of smell

* digestive problems

* irritable bowel

* heartburn and reflux

* respiratory infections, including sinus infections, bronchitis, and pneumonia

* shortness of breath

* chest pain

* painful intercourse for women

* frequent urinary infections

* brittle nails and nails with ridges

Other Symptoms

For many of us, Sjögren's syndrome is much more than dryness, and sometimes we wonder why so much of the concern centers on dryness when other symptoms cause the most trouble. These "other symptoms" often complicate the diagnostic picture by being characteristic of a number of different disorders, as well as other autoimmune diseases. Many physicians and dentists identify Sjögren's syndrome with dryness, so, if a patient doesn't clearly exhibit this symptom, they often don't recognize Sjögren's, or don't see the symptoms as interrelated. Sometimes the dryness that is classic for Sjögren's appears suddenly. Usually, however, dryness develops so slowly that patients and their doctors don't recognize it early in the disease process. Without easy-to-diagnose dryness, doctors can miss other symptoms that might lead to a diagnosis of Sjögren's.

Knowing about potential symptoms can be a mixed blessing. As authors, we chose to provide all the information we felt you might need. You will want to know if symptoms you have might be connected to your Sjögren's, and if you are familiar with other symptoms before they appear, you will recognize them and not be frightened by them. It's also important to secure the support and understanding of your family and friends by letting them know the potential complications of this disease and how difficult living with Sjögren's syndrome can be.

We have included a list of the many diverse and seemingly unrelated symptoms someone with Sjögren's might experience. Other symptoms are also covered in chapter 4. While possible symptoms of Sjögren's are listed here, keep in mind that you might not develop *any* of these.

Other Possible Symptoms

* muscle and joint pain, stiffness (especially in the morning)

* swollen parotid glands (the salivary glands just in front of the ears that swell when one has the mumps)

* swollen submandibular glands (the salivary glands just under your jaw line)

* fatigue

* low-grade fevers
* numbness, tingling, or change in sensation (especially in the feet, legs, hands, or arms)
* facial numbness
* nerve pain
* increased symptoms or "flare" during or immediately following pregnancy
* irritable bowel
* nausea
* hives
* small red spots on legs (petechiae)
* red or purple spots on legs that look like bruises (bleeding in the skin, or purpura)
* muscle weakness
* skin ulcers
* burning and/or painful feet
* fingers that turn white, blue, and red in response to cold temperatures (called "Raynaud's phenomenon)
* hair loss
* hearing loss
* esophageal spasms
* esophageal "webbing" (webs of tissue that narrow the esophagus and increase problems with swallowing)
* frequent or painful urination
* difficulty sleeping
* dizziness
* concentration and memory problems

We've listed a lot of symptoms, and you might now have more questions than when you started reading! Most of us share common questions about living with Sjögren's syndrome and what our future might hold. Remember: you are not alone! Here are a few questions you might have:

* **If I have Sjögren's syndrome, will I have all of these symptoms?**

   No! Remember that everyone is different. These are just many of the symptoms that can be connected with Sjögren's.

* **If I have some of these symptoms, does this mean I have Sjögren's syndrome?**

   No! These symptoms are common with many different disorders.

* **If I have Sjögren's and later develop one of these symptoms, does this necessarily mean the symptom is caused by the Sjögren's?**

   No. That's why it's important to see your doctor, who can determine if the symptom is connected to your Sjögren's syndrome or is unrelated.

What's in a Name?

Disease names help categorize diseases. In the 1960s, two terms came into use to describe Sjögren's syndrome—*primary* and *secondary*—and many doctors still use these terms today.

As we've mentioned, you can be diagnosed with one, or more than one, autoimmune disease. If you have Sjögren's syndrome and cannot be diagnosed with another, major autoimmune disease, you might be said to have primary Sjögren's syndrome. If you are diagnosed with Sjögren's in addition to another, major autoimmune disease, such as rheumatoid arthritis, lupus, or scleroderma, then your Sjögren's might be called secondary Sjögren's syndrome.

There is a growing trend in the medical world to drop this differentiation, and many specialists do not label the Sjögren's differently depending on how many autoimmune diseases you have. In fact, primary Sjögren's patients are likely to develop additional autoimmune disorders. Some specialists speak of an "overlap disease," which is when you have Sjögren's syndrome and a strong indication of another autoimmune disease but the latter cannot be definitely proven.

Who Gets Sjögren's Syndrome?

Nine out of ten of those diagnosed with Sjögren's syndrome are women, and most are age forty-five and older. However, anyone can have Sjögren's, including men and children. Nor does Sjögren's discriminate among different racial and ethnic groups. Autoimmune diseases tend to run in families, so there could be several different autoimmune diseases in your family tree. Because recognition and diagnosis of autoimmune diseases have made great progress only in recent years, it's sometimes difficult to know if someone in generations before you had an autoimmune disease.

Why do more women than men get autoimmune diseases? No clear answer has been found, but there are two theories. First, we know that many women are diagnosed at times of great hormonal change, such as during pregnancy, following the birth of a child, or upon menopause. Because female hormones can make the disease worse, scientists theorize this is why women are more susceptible. A second theory notes that women's immune systems are more complex than men's, because they are designed to allow a baby to grow and develop and not attack it as a foreign entity. The more complex something is, the more things there are that can go wrong!

We need many more studies on Sjögren's syndrome to obtain definitive statistics, especially about age. While more people are diagnosed after age forty-five, this could mean that most women don't develop Sjögren's until later in life, but it might also be that medical professionals do not recognize the disease when it appears in younger people. Dry mouth and dry eyes are hallmark symptoms of Sjögren's and are relatively easy to measure and recognize compared to other, less obvious symptoms. But many people do not suffer severely enough from dryness to recognize it until they get older. We often take more medications as we age, and side effects frequently aggravate dryness so that we finally complain. Dryness due directly to Sjögren's can grow worse with time; chronic inflammation and damage to moisture-producing glands usually take place over a long period. Finally, dryness worsens with the onset of menopause.

When doctors are trained to look for Sjögren's syndrome in older women, they are more likely to diagnose it in their older female patients.

Disease Patterns and Flares

Symptoms can wax and wane. Some days you will feel less dry than other days. Many factors can contribute to this effect. Inflammation comes and goes depending on how active your disease is at a given time. Some medications can increase dryness, so when you stop these medications, dryness decreases. Some foods increase dryness, a major culprit being caffeine, so if your mouth or eyes are particularly bothersome, skip the coffee and tea! Dry air and wind can contribute to dryness. Stress, fatigue, and lack of sleep make symptoms worse for any disease, and Sjögren's is no exception.

Many people from time to time refer to having a disease flare, which means an exacerbation of their usual symptoms. Flares can be intense; at other times, many of the symptoms might remit or give you peace for a while. With Sjögren's, you often feel like you're suffering from a low-grade flu, but rather than tell friends and family your litany of symptoms, you may simply say you're feeling much more "Sjögren-y" today!

Possible Causes

Scientists believe development of Sjögren's involves a complex gene-environment interaction. The common understanding is that you inherit a genetic tendency to develop an autoimmune disease, and something from your surroundings or environment triggers the disease.

Sjögren's syndrome is not caused by one gene. Everyone inherits many genetic markers, and specific markers are found more frequently in those who develop Sjögren's syndrome than those who don't. Genetic markers most often associated with autoimmune disease and Sjögren's are called "HLA," which stands for human leukocyte antigen. An antigen is a protein that reacts with an antibody. Letters and numbers added after the "HLA" indicate specific genes. Certain HLA-DR markers, particularly HLA-DRw52 and HLA-DR3, are frequently associated with Sjögren's. HLA-DR4 (there are many HLA-DR markers) has been identified with Sjögren's when accompanied by rheumatoid arthritis. HLA-DQ and HLA-DP markers also have been associated with Sjögren's. Probably, several markers found together make you more likely to develop certain autoimmune diseases. Unfortunately, there is no simple answer. Genetics is a complex field, but more is being learned and understood all the time.

Triggers are usually termed "environmental." This means that something in your environment starts the autoimmune process that ultimately becomes an autoimmune disease. A virus or bacteria could be the environmental trigger. Unidentified viruses or bacteria are suspected in Sjögren's syndrome as well as lupus, rheumatoid arthritis, and multiple sclerosis. Other potential environmental triggers include chemical exposure, drugs, foods, and hormones found in meat (Hess 1999).

While we don't know for certain what causes Sjögren's syndrome, scientists have discovered that certain environmental exposures have caused or are highly suspected of causing other autoimmune diseases or related conditions. For example, a specific bacteria is suspected in the autoimmune Crohn's disease, which affects the intestine; *C. trachomatis* is being investigated in reactive arthritis, sometimes called Reiter's syndrome; and Coxsackie virus might be involved in autoimmune diabetes. The bacteria *Borrelia burgdorferi* found in a tick causes Lyme disease, and another bacteria was discovered to cause Whipple's disease, an arthritis and malabsorption disorder. Group A *Streptococcus* and *Staphylococcus aureus*, more commonly known as strep throat and staph infections, are suspects in the progression of some diseases, and Hepatitis B and Hepatitis C viruses are possibly causes or exacerbators of vasculitis, which is inflammation of the blood vessels found in many autoimmune disorders. Recent studies show that human herpes virus 6 might play a role in the development of multiple sclerosis.

Modern life has brought pesticides, industrial waste, and chemical additives and the addition of hormones to food and drug production. Many of these have been connected with autoimmune symptoms. While none have been directly shown to induce Sjögren's syndrome, large doses from occupational exposures are suspected of playing a major role in the development of other autoimmune diseases. Chemicals considered to have such a role include mercury, silica, and vinyl chloride (Parks, Conrad, and Cooper 1999). Mercury fillings in teeth have been studied and found *not* to cause autoimmune symptoms.

Estrogen and estrogenic compounds (especially estradiol) can alter the immune system and predispose one to autoimmune disease (Ahmed et al. 1999). Other examples of possible culprits include the sleep aid L-tryptophan (Takagi et al. 1995) and adulterated rapeseed oils. Ultraviolet radiation can also be harmful. In addition, exposure during pregnancy to environmental agents might predispose a fetus to develop autoimmune disease later in life (Holladay 1999). Auto-immunity can continue long after the trigger has disappeared, making it difficult to pinpoint an exact cause.

We know we've just presented you with some complicated terms and ideas, but we want to make the point that there are many scientific studies connecting autoimmune disease to environmental agents. While none has yet been linked directly to Sjögren's syndrome, the fact that environmental influences have been linked directly to other autoimmune disorders leads scientists to believe that it is likely that links will also be found with Sjögren's. Regardless of the exposure, however, your genetic makeup most likely determines whether you do or do not have an autoimmune reaction to a virus, bacteria, or other environmental exposure.

Your Immune System

Let's take a look at how the immune system works to defend the body from foreign invaders. The immune system includes a type of white blood cells called lymphocytes, lymph nodes or glands, and lymph tissue, including the thymus and spleen.

Two major lymphocytes are T cells and B cells. Immune cells develop in the bone marrow from stem cells. T cells develop from immune cells that move to the thymus, which is located just below the neck and in the center of the chest, and it is here that they develop the means to distinguish between "self" and "nonself," or that which is a normal part of your body and that which is foreign. They remember what is foreign and what is not. T cells, then, oversee the immune system, telling the other immune cells, such as B cells, what to do. B cells develop from immune cells that move from the bone marrow to the lymph nodes, which are located all over the body; you're probably most familiar with those in the neck, armpits, and groin because you can sometimes feel these nodes swell during a local or general infection. These areas swell during increased production of antibodies to fight infection.

Other white blood cells that identify and destroy foreign substances include macrophages, neutrophils, and natural killer cells. Macrophages and neutrophils engulf foreign antigens, such as bacteria, and destroy them by producing toxic molecules. In autoimmune diseases, production of these toxic molecules can continue unchecked to inflame and damage surrounding tissue. Natural killer cells can identify and destroy foreign substances without having previously encountered those substances. Some lymphocytes signal T cells and B cells that an infection is present.

Other terms that you might hear about in relation to immune function and the development of autoimmune disease are *complement,* a component of T cells called *MHC,* and *cytokines. Complement* is a group of proteins in the blood that bind to immune complexes in some types of inflammation. If complement is low, then inflammation may be greater. MHC, or major histocompatibility complexes, are molecules on the surface of T cells and most other cells, and have a part in recognition of self versus nonself. MHCs on a T cell and another cell interact, helping the T cell recognize the other cell. Finally, when the MHCs interact, T cells secrete cytokines, proteins that signal other T cells and cause other cells to grow, become active, or die.

The immune system does not always function correctly and can thus cause inflammation and even attack body organs and produce antibodies that damage tissue. Cytokines can contribute to inflammation. Antibodies might gather inappropriately at a particular site in the body, binding together into immune complexes and causing inflammation, resulting in many autoimmune disease symptoms and complications.

In addition, B cells can mistakenly identify your own tissue as a foreign invader and destroy that tissue. This can happen with the moisture-producing exocrine glands in Sjögren's syndrome, preventing the production of adequate moisture. Inflammation and destruction can happen anywhere in the body. For example, vasculitis, or inflammation in the small blood vessels, can block nourishment and damage surrounding tissue.

Interestingly, you can have normal tissue in the salivary glands, yet those glands still may not produce saliva. Another way of looking at it is that saliva production can continue to decrease over time, even though the glands are not suffering increased damage. This leads scientists to think something in addition to the damage and inflammation must be causing the dysfunction.

A small degree of autoimmunity is actually normal. When auto-immunity becomes out of control, autoimmune disease develops.

Finally, here are some additional frequently asked questions pertinent to understanding "What is Sjögren's syndrome?"

How will having Sjögren's affect your life? This is one of the most complicated questions to answer, so we'll just say that it depends. You will have to get to know your own body, learn about your disease, and work on ways to deal with your symptoms and how they will fit into your life. It's different for everyone, but we hope this book will provide the knowledge and tools and positive outlook to make your life easier. Will your life change? Definitely! Will it change for the worse? We would say that it will simply be different, and you will need to learn to prioritize and experiment with the best ways to meet your particular challenges. Relationships and life will change, but we hope that you will find ways to accept and cope with those circumstances you cannot change, and ultimately use your illness to increase your enjoyment and appreciation of life.

Is Sjögren's syndrome contagious? No. You cannot catch Sjögren's from someone else, and they cannot catch it from you. Sadly, some people who do not know any better fear eating from the same dishes as someone with a chronic illness like Sjögren's syndrome. We'll say it again: You *cannot* catch Sjögren's syndrome.

Can you inherit Sjögren's syndrome? No, you do not directly inherit autoimmune disease, although you might inherit the susceptibility to developing autoimmune disease. Autoimmune diseases tend to cluster in families, although family members often express autoimmune disease differently. For example, a great-aunt might have had rheumatoid arthritis, a cousin, lupus, and you have Sjögren's syndrome. Because these diseases overlap, you might also have more than one disease or your symptoms might cross the spectrum of more than one disease.

What did you do to develop Sjögren's? Nothing. You are not responsible for having your disease. Your genetic makeup proba-bly made your immune system susceptible to reacting to an outside agent—perhaps a common, perhaps a not-so-common, virus or environmental exposure. Until researchers' understanding increases, we don't know how to avoid getting the disease, and we don't have vaccines to prevent it.

Can you have children? What are the risks? Yes, you can have children. You need to be monitored during pregnancy, because certain autoantibodies that are common in Sjögren's syndrome can cause fetal heart block. Your chances of heart block are one in twenty if you've never had a child with heart block and are positive for these antibodies. We'll discuss heart block in more detail in chapter 4. You can also experience major flares with the hormone changes of pregnancy, but you might instead feel much better during pregnancy; it will vary from person to person and with each pregnancy in the same person. If fatigue is a problem with your disease, then be prepared for the added fatigue of having a newborn. If you can arrange for help, do so!

Is Sjögren's syndrome serious? Yes! Just look at all the possible symptoms we have listed. You'll learn in this book about possible consequences on quality of life, work, and relationships, and about the body organs and systems affected, from the risk of lymphoma (about 5 percent) to risks during pregnancy. But, you'll also learn some positive steps you can take to deal with the effects of Sjögren's syndrome on your world.

Can you die from this disease? The vast majority of people with Sjögren's will live long and productive lives. Being diagnosed with Sjögren's syndrome does not mean your life has come to an end. While quality of life can be impaired, you can find ways to accommodate your illness, make symptoms better, and prevent serious complications. Sometimes, though, serious complications do occur. Sjögren's syndrome is sometimes called the "crossover disease," meaning that it can become malignant and advance to lymphoma. This progression is rare, but because it can happen, it's important to be monitored regularly by your doctor. Problems of the central nervous system, also a rare complication, need immediate attention. Finally, because you can develop multiple autoimmune diseases, with Sjögren's syndrome, you must understand the need to remain under a knowledgeable doctor's care.

What We Know Now

Many research studies are needed on Sjögren's syndrome before we fully understand this disease. We don't have the statistics to tell us exactly how many people have which symptoms, or who is more likely to develop a particular complication. Our definition and treatment of Sjögren's will surely change as we learn more.

Let's summarize briefly what we *do* know. We know that Sjögren's syndrome is an autoimmune disease. Sjögren's targets the moisture-producing glands, but it can affect any body organ or system and result in a wide spectrum of symptoms for the individual. It's a prevalent disease, affecting as many as four million Americans and many more worldwide. It strikes all races and ethnic groups equally, but it strikes women more than men at a ratio of nine to one. Sjögren's syndrome is a serious disease, with serious consequences, and it deserves serious attention from medical, dental, and allied professional schools, practicing professionals, and researchers.

2

What Makes Up
a Diagnosis?

Correct diagnosis is critical if you have Sjögren's syndrome so that you can obtain the proper treatment, prevent complications, and recognize problems as they arise. A diagnosis also provides a label enabling physicians, health care workers, and friends and family to understand and more appropriately respond to your experience. Unfortunately, the correct diagnosis of Sjögren's syndrome often requires a long, frustrating, and arduous process. Some with Sjögren's have a sudden onset of symptoms and visit a medical specialist who recognizes the possibility of Sjögren's and immediately investigates it as the cause, but for most people, this scenario is not typical. It often takes years, not weeks, for symptoms to become recognizable as a pattern, to be seen as interrelated, and for a patient to be tested and to establish positive results that help a medical professional arrive at the correct diagnosis.

The Not-So-Simple Diagnosis

A recent study found that it took slightly more than six years for the average Sjögren's syndrome patient to obtain a diagnosis (Boston Healthcare Associates 1996). Why so long?

First of all, there is no one single test that can determine whether you have Sjögren's. A combination of tests, examinations, and questions are necessary to make the diagnosis. Furthermore, the first doctor you see may not be knowledgeable about Sjögren's syndrome. Different medical specialists might be approached for one or more of many different symptoms, and unless a specialist is trained and experienced in mapping the interconnection of those symptoms, or even knows to ask about symptoms outside his or her medical field, achieving a correct diagnosis becomes more complicated. For example, a dentist might treat your rampant caries (cavities) that occur as a result of dry mouth without delving further into the potential cause of the destruction.

And what if you don't have any obvious dryness? The diagnosis gets even more difficult. For example, if you visit a neurologist for numbness in your feet or legs, the neurologist most likely will not see signs of major neurological complications or damage, and you might leave with only your mental health being questioned. Most neurologists are not trained to connect a sensation of numbness with joint and muscle pain or swollen salivary glands or recurring eye infections. The neurologist won't ask about those symptoms, and if you aren't aware of the possible symptoms of Sjögren's, you won't think of them either.

Who Makes the Diagnosis?

Usually a rheumatologist, dentist, or ophthalmologist will initially diagnose Sjögren's syndrome. This triad of specialists diagnoses and treats the most common symptoms of Sjögren's. The rheumatologist is best equipped to oversee a complete workup, check the systemic aspects, and recommend other specialists as needed. A rheumatologist specializes in rheumatic, connective tissue disease and arthritis-related diseases and is the specialist most likely to know about Sjögren's. He or she can make a diagnosis based on a combination of a physical exam, medical history, lab tests, and responses to questions about present-day symptoms and activities. Most likely, however, you will not see a rheumatologist until a connective tissue disease is suspected. That referral could come from the family physician, dentist, ophthalmologist, or any health professional who recognizes symptoms related to Sjögren's. Many people give up until they develop those symptoms most easily linked with Sjögren's.

Getting the Picture

A rheumatologist would first take down your medical history and list of current symptoms and ask questions to help determine the diagnosis and rule out other disorders. Questions would include those about the medical history of family members and about medications you take. Then he or she would do a physical exam, looking for manifestations of dryness, vasculitis, and joint swelling, measuring muscle strength, and checking lungs and heart. Finally, a doctor will have blood tests done by a lab.

When the dentist, other oral health care specialist, or ophthalmologist is visited, they will run tests specific to their medical areas as well.

What Tests Might You Expect?

Your rheumatologist might run some of the following blood tests:

* **Antinuclear antibody, or ANA, test.** In Sjögren's syndrome, certain antibodies react to the self, or your own body, and are called autoantibodies. The rheumatologist looks for these autoantibodies when diagnosing someone suspected of having Sjögren's syndrome. About 70 percent of those with Sjögren's have a positive ANA.

    ANAs are traditionally reported in *titers*. The first number is always one, and a positive test result means the second number is higher than forty or eighty. For example, a titer of 1:320 is considered positive. A higher titer, however, does not provide a reliable gauge for judging severity of symptoms or disease. A positive ANA is not proof that a person has Sjögren's syndrome. This finding is associated with many rheumatic diseases.

A new version of this test now rates the ANA from 1 to 12, with 12 being the highest and correlating to a titer of 1:1280.

Specific autoantibodies identified with Sjögren's include anti-SSA and anti-SSB. In Sjögren's syndrome, 70 percent of patients are positive for SSA and 40 percent are positive for SSB.

* **Other autoantibodies tests.** A doctor might test for other specific autoantibodies to help rule out other auto-immune diseases. SSA and SSB are most prevalent in Sjögren's patients but are also found in lupus patients who are not diagnosed with Sjögren's. The doctor can look for autoantibodies associated with other specific diseases.

* **Rheumatoid factor (RF).** This antibody test is a general indicator of rheumatic disease but is not specific. Sixty to seventy percent of Sjögren's syndrome patients test positive for RF.

* **Erythrocyte sedimentation rate (ESR or "sed rate").** The ESR test measures inflammation. A positive sed rate can occur in any illness from the flu to autoimmune disease. Because Sjögren's syndrome involves inflammation, the ESR is simply one more test that will help complete the diagnostic picture.

The sed rate is measured in numbers, with a higher number indicating greater inflammation. Traditionally, any number greater than twenty was considered an elevated sed rate, but increasingly, physicians and researchers consider numbers only over forty as significant.

* **Serum protein electrophoresis.** Immunoglobulins, or Igs, are normal blood proteins or antibodies, and they are usually elevated in Sjögren's syndrome. The different kinds of immunoglobulins will be reported as IgG, IgM, and IgA (or immunoglobulin G, immunoglobulin M, and immuno-globulin A). The test might be repeated from time to time to monitor disease activity.

Ophthalmologists might perform the following tests for dry eyes:

* **Schirmer test.** This standard test for dry eye involves placing small strips of filter paper between the lower eyelid and eyeball. After five minutes, the amount of wetting on the strips is measured, giving a rough estimate of tear production for each eye. Results will vary depending on whether an anesthetic is used, and ophthalmologists differ in their preference. A low value (less than five to ten millimeters of wetting) is suggestive but not diagnostic of dry eye.

* **Staining.** Special dyes allow the ophthalmologist to observe abnormal cells on the surface of the eye. The most common dyes are rose bengal and lissamine green. Lissamine green is used more frequently now in the United States and appears to be less uncomfortable for patients.

* **Slit lamp exam.** Tears seen on the lower eyelid through this magnifying instrument can help the ophthalmologist assess tear volume. Tears are measured when the eye is in a resting or unstimulated state, in contrast to the Schirmer test, which can stimulate tear production. The slit lamp exam can also show if there is inflammation of the eye.

A dentist or otolaryngologist might perform the following tests:

* **Lip biopsy.** This procedure is used to confirm lymphocytic infiltration into the minor salivary glands and is one of the most definitive tests for Sjögren's syndrome. Such infiltration destroys salivary gland function.

    The procedure to remove minor salivary glands has improved greatly in the last few years. Now, only a small incision is made on the inside surface of your lower lip and minor salivary glands are individually removed. The tissue is examined under a microscope.

    Even with recent improvements in the procedure, you should always insist that the practitioner performing the biopsy has done many procedures before; it's a simple process, but there are many minor nerves that can be nicked if someone is inexperienced. Biopsy of major salivary glands is rarely if ever done because major facial nerves run next to these glands.

The lip biopsy is scored according to damage to the salivary gland. Twelve is the highest score, indicating the greatest damage. A score higher than one is considered positive for damage and a positive indicator of Sjögren's, yet normal patients who don't have Sjögren's have been known to have scores greater than one.

* **Salivary gland flow.** This process measures the amount of saliva by providing a quantitative measure of saliva over a specific time period. The normal parotid gland flow rate is 1.5 milliliters per fifteen minutes. In Sjögren's syndrome, flow rate is lower.

* **Salivary scintigraphy.** Salivary gland function is measured by this test after low-level radioactive material is injected into a vein. Saliva in the salivary glands and mouth takes up the radioactivity and can be seen and measured. In Sjögren's, little or no saliva will be visible.

* **Sialography.** Your salivary duct system can be visualized clearly by the sialography after radiologically sensitive dye is injected into your salivary duct system. Because it relies heavily on observer skills, the sialography is not a reliable diagnostic tool for Sjögren's (Spijkervet et al. 2002), but it can still provide important information. An abnormal pattern is produced by the inflammation common to Sjögren's, so this observation is useful. The sialography can also show if an obstruction unrelated to Sjögren's is causing your dry mouth.

Other tests rheumatologists might perform include:

* **Urinalysis.** A urinalysis will be used to check for kidney inflammation.

* **Thyroid function tests.** Because autoimmune thyroid disease is prevalent and can accompany Sjögren's, your physician will want to make sure your thyroid is functioning normally.

* **Liver function tests.** Liver function tests can be abnormal in Sjögren's. Sometimes this finding will simply be something your physician will want to monitor and is not

cause for alarm. Your physician can determine if the test results indicate liver complications that might be related to Sjögren's.

* **Chest X ray.** A chest X ray might be done to check for signs of inflammation in the lungs.

Basic tests for diagnosis are handled by a rheumatologist, dentist, and ophthalmologist. However, you might need to see other specialists for testing and treatment of other specific symptoms. For example, if you tell your rheumatologist that you experience a great deal of numbness and pain in your extremities, and that medications are not helping, you might be sent to a neurologist for further testing.

When Lab Results Are Inconclusive

Sometimes you will have symptoms that indicate a diagnosis of Sjögren's syndrome, but the lab tests are negative or inconclusive. What happens then? Your physician might label you as having "possible" or "probable" Sjögren's or other undifferentiated (meaning it can't be determined accurately) connective tissue or autoimmune disease and wait to see what develops. In the meantime, you should be treated for the symptoms, and tests should be repeated from time to time.

Although a clear majority (70 percent) of Sjögren's syndrome patients are positive for the SSA autoimmune antibody test, 30 percent of patients with Sjögren's are not positive. If you test negative for the SSA antibody, it does not rule out a diagnosis of Sjögren's.

Different results for lab tests might be obtained depending on the lab your doctor uses. The lack of uniformity among labs should be considered if there is a question about your lab results.

Exclusion of Other Causes

Sjögren's syndrome mimics many other disorders, so part of the physician's job of diagnosis entails ruling out other causes for your symptoms. Allergies can cause many of the presenting symptoms (the first recognizable symptoms) of Sjögren's, including red, itchy, irritated eyes, scratchy sore throat, and stuffy nasal passages. In both allergies and autoimmune disease, there is an overproduction of antibodies. In Sjögren's, a surplus of antibodies is produced because your immune system reacts to your own tissues as if they were foreign, while in allergies a surplus of antibodies is produced in reaction to a foreign substance that is not normally threatening. Someone with Sjögren's can also have allergies.

Similar neurological symptoms are found in many autoimmune disorders or as initial symptoms of unrelated diseases such as Lou Gehrig's disease, also known as amyotrophic lateral sclerosis, or ALS. Sjögren's patients can be initially misdiagnosed as having multiple sclerosis. Some researchers believe you can have both Sjögren's and multiple sclerosis, just as you can have Sjögren's and lupus or Sjögren's and rheumatoid arthritis, while others believe that once you have a confirmed diagnosis of Sjögren's, neurological symptoms can be attributed to Sjögren's, no matter how severe they become.

Many medications can cause or exacerbate dryness symptoms. Aching joints and muscles can be caused by osteoarthritis, as well as by many of the autoimmune and connective tissue disorders. Fatigue can be traced to a multitude of potential sources. Hepatitis C causes Sjögren's-like symptoms and must be ruled out for a diagnosis of Sjögren's.

Diagnostic Differences

Physicians diagnosing Sjögren's syndrome have lacked a clear and universally accepted definition of the disease, often resulting in frustration for patients and doctors alike. Because different sets of criteria might be used to determine if someone has Sjögren's, you might be diagnosed with Sjögren's by one doctor but would not under different criteria used by someone else. There have been national and regional differences in diagnostic guidelines.

We still need universally accepted diagnostic criteria for the clinician to use, and the Sjögren's Syndrome Foundation is working to ensure that such criteria will be developed. We have made some progress. For the first time ever, researchers worldwide have agreed upon a set of criteria for determining if you have Sjögren's syndrome. The "International Classification Criteria for Sjögren's Syndrome," initiated and sponsored by the Sjögren's Syndrome Foundation, was designed for uniform diagnosis of Sjögren's in clinical studies, or studies to test treatment options for patients (Vitali et al. 2002). These guidelines for deciding whether or not you have

Sjögren's are probably stricter than the guidelines your own physician will use, because they were designed with research in mind.

What these strict criteria do represent is a yardstick by which it is possible to measure the most basic, definitive diagnosis for Sjögren's syndrome. If you fit the criteria, you definitely have Sjögren's syndrome. If you don't fit the criteria, you *might* have Sjögren's, and your physician can then use his or her knowledge and experience to decide whether or not you do.

Strict Criteria for Sjögren's

The "International Classification Criteria for Sjögren's Syndrome" set guidelines for diagnosing primary and secondary Sjögren's syndrome. The guidelines are divided into subjective criteria, meaning symptoms that you feel and recognize but that can't be measured by a lab test, and objective criteria, or tests that can be scientifically measured.

According to these criteria, for diagnosis of primary Sjögren's syndrome you must have:

* no additional major, connective tissue disease, *plus either*

* four of the six criteria included under subjective and objective criteria listed below, *plus* positive results for a lip biopsy or for autoantibodies, *or*

* three out of four of the objective criteria.

To diagnose secondary Sjögren's syndrome, you must have:

* the presence of another major, connective tissue disease, *plus*

* either eye or mouth symptoms listed under the subjective criteria, *plus*

* positive results for two out of three of the first three objective criteria, meaning that you are positive for two of the following: ocular tests, lip biopsy, or salivary gland involvement.

Subjective Criteria

Ocular symptoms. You must have a positive response to at least one of the following questions:

1. Have you had daily, persistent, troublesome dry eyes for more than three months?

2. Do you have a recurrent sensation of sand in the eyes?

3. Do you use tear substitutes more than three times a day?

Oral symptoms. You must have a positive response to at least one of the following questions:

1. Have you had a daily feeling of dry mouth for more than three months?

2. Have you had recurrently or persistently swollen salivary glands as an adult?

3. Do you frequently drink liquids to aid in swallowing dry food?

Objective Criteria

Ocular signs. You must have a positive result for at least one of the following two tests:

1. Schirmer test, performed without anesthesia (less than or equal to five millimeters in five minutes)

2. Rose bengal or lissamine green dye score of four or more

Histopathology. You must have a positive lip biopsy.

Salivary gland involvement. You must have a positive result for at least one of the following three tests:

1. Unstimulated whole salivary flow (1.5 milliliters or less in fifteen minutes)

2. Parotid sialography

3. Salivary scintigraphy

Autoantibodies. Antibodies to either SSA (Ro) or SSB (La) antigens, or both, must be present in your blood.

Finally, the criteria state that you cannot be diagnosed with Sjögren's syndrome if you have had specific preexisting conditions. These include:

* past head and neck radiation therapy

* hepatitis C infection

* AIDS, or acquired immunodeficiency disease

* preexisting lymphoma

* sarcoidosis

* graft-versus-host disease, a condition that sometimes occurs following bone marrow transplants

* use of anticholinergic drugs (used to relieve cramping and spasms of the stomach, intestines, and bladder, and sometimes used for severe menstrual cramping)

Related and Overlapping Diseases

Autoimmune diseases are related and share similar mechanisms. Therefore, it is not surprising that you can have multiple or overlapping autoimmune disorders. Many autoimmune diseases are target-specific, meaning one organ or system is targeted by the autoantibodies. For example, in autoimmune thyroid disease, autoantibodies attack the thyroid. In autoimmune liver disease, autoantibodies attack the liver.

If a person produces antibodies against one target, it is not impossible to produce them against additional targets. While autoantibodies attack the moisture-producing glands in Sjögren's syndrome, they can also attack any body organ or system. This process might be considered part of Sjögren's, or someone with Sjögren's syndrome might be described as having multiple autoimmune disorders. Regardless of how the disorders are labeled, once your physician suspects you have autoimmune disease, the treatment will largely depend on the symptoms.

About half of those with Sjögren's syndrome have another diagnosed major autoimmune disorder, and many have overlapping disorders or symptoms of other disorders. The most common disorder found in Sjögren's syndrome patients is autoimmune thyroid. Also common are rheumatoid arthritis, lupus, scleroderma, and fibromyalgia. Someone with Sjögren's can have any or several of the more-than-eighty other autoimmune disorders along with their Sjögren's syndrome.

Let's take a look at what some of those disorders may be.

Autoimmune thyroid disorders. There are two kinds of autoimmune thyroid disease: Graves' disease and Hashimoto's thyroiditis. Graves' disease involves a hyper, or overactive, thyroid. In Hashimoto's thyroiditis the thyroid is underactive.

Rheumatoid arthritis. This is a connective tissue, autoimmune disease that causes joint inflammation, swelling, and sometimes damage to the joints. Joint pain and stiffness, especially in the morning, are common. Rheumatoid arthritis can affect any body organ and system.

Systemic lupus erythematosis (or lupus). This autoimmune disease is closely related to Sjögren's syndrome genetically. Sometimes a person with lupus will later develop Sjögren's, or less frequently, someone with Sjögren's might develop lupus, or have symptoms indicative of lupus that do not quite meet the lupus criteria. Lupus can attack any body organ or system. A butterfly rash over the nose and cheeks is a classic symptom of lupus, although a majority of those with lupus do not have this symptom. Major complications of lupus can include kidney and neurological problems.

Scleroderma. *Scleroderma* literally means "hardening of the skin." Local scleroderma affects the skin alone, while the systemic form of scleroderma, sometimes called systemic sclerosis, can affect any organ in the body. The connective tissue loses its elasticity and ability to function. The skin becomes tightly stretched instead of remaining supple, and patients can find it difficult to have full joint movement or even to eat. When scleroderma affects the internal organs, such as the heart, lungs, and gastrointestinal tract, those organs do not function properly.

Multiple sclerosis. Multiple sclerosis is believed by most researchers to be an autoimmune disease. It affects the central nervous system, causing symptoms ranging from mild numbness and tingling to paralysis.

Inflammatory bowel disease. Inflammatory bowel diseases include Crohn's and ulcerative colitis. They are believed to be autoimmune diseases causing inflammation of the gastrointestinal tract.

Crohn's can affect any part of the digestive tract, whereas ulcerative colitis affects only the colon, or large intestine. Symptoms of both disorders include abdominal pain, diarrhea, and sometimes rectal bleeding. Inflammatory bowel diseases are not directly related to irritable bowel syndrome or spastic colon.

Raynaud's disease. In Raynaud's, blood flow does not get to the fingers or toes, and they turn white, blue, and then red upon exposure to the cold. A patient can have Raynaud's alone or with another autoimmune disease, such as Sjögren's syndrome, scleroderma, or lupus. Raynaud's can be associated with vasculitis, or inflammation of the blood vessels.

The severity of the symptoms defines whether you have Raynaud's disease or Raynaud's phenomenon. "Phenomenon" is used when the Raynaud's causes color changes and pain. "Disease" is used when fingers and toes are actually damaged, potentially leading to gangrene or other complications.

Antiphospholipid syndrome. Antiphospholipid syndrome is an autoimmune condition in which antibodies are made against phospholipids in your body, resulting in an increased tendency to form blood clots. Antiphospholipid syndrome can cause second trimester miscarriage. Sjögren's syndrome and other autoimmune disease patients can have this condition.

Interstitial cystitis. The bladder is chronically inflamed in interstitial cystitis, causing frequent and painful urination. While not generally considered to be an autoimmune disorder, it can occur frequently in Sjögren's and other autoimmune patients.

Myositis. Myositis is a broad term meaning inflammation of the muscles. Different forms of myositis include polymyositis and dermatomyositis, which are thought to be autoimmune diseases. Myositis can accompany Sjögren's syndrome and frequently results in muscle weakness. Blood tests often show high levels of muscle enzymes. Usually an electromyography (EMG) and muscle biopsy are done to confirm the diagnosis.

Autoimmune liver disease. Autoimmune liver disease can occur either on its own or with another autoimmune disease such as Sjögren's syndrome. There are two types of autoimmune liver disease. Primary biliary cirrhosis more frequently occurs with Sjögren's and damages the liver's bile ducts. Often there are no symptoms, and it is discovered through liver function blood tests. Autoimmune hepatitis involves inflammation of the liver. Common symptoms are jaundice, aching joints, itching, and fatigue.

Alopecia areata. Alopecia is defined as the loss of hair and can occur with many autoimmune diseases, including Sjögren's syndrome. Alopecia areata is an autoimmune disease resulting in hair loss, including hair on the scalp, eyebrows, eyelashes, and elsewhere on the body.

Myasthenia gravis. Myasthenia gravis is an autoimmune disease characterized by muscular weakness. Neurological signals are not transmitted correctly to affected muscles. Sometimes the eyes alone are affected, but myasthenia gravis can impact any muscle.

Ménière's disease. Ménière's disease affects the ear, causing loss of balance and potential hearing loss. Ringing in the ears (tinnitus) and dizziness and vertigo are common symptoms. It is most likely an autoimmune disease.

Fibromyalgia. Little is known about the cause of this painful disorder. Many researchers do not regard it to be an autoimmune disease while others suspect that it might be. It is characterized by widespread muscular pain and specific tender points on the surface of the body. It may occur alone or together with autoimmune diseases and frequently coexists with Sjögren's syndrome.

As we have said, Sjögren's syndrome can mimic other disorders, its symptoms can appear unrelated, and patients are often misdiagnosed and go undiagnosed. Though doctors' ability to diagnose Sjögren's is improving, diagnosis largely remains an art. Better education of all medical and allied health professionals is desperately needed to improve chances for a proper diagnosis, and, subsequently, early and proper treatment. Increased research is needed so that better and more sensitive tests for Sjögren's can be developed.

3

How Do You
Treat Sjögren's?

Sjögren's syndrome is a chronic illness, but there are many things
you can do to deal with your symptoms in order to feel better, prevent complications, and improve your quality of life. We believe that
learning as much as possible about your illness will help you and
your doctor decide on the best course of treatment, improve the
chances that you will follow that treatment, and ultimately improve
the outcome. By reading this book and pursuing additional resources
for support and information, you are already on the road to a sound
treatment plan.

   The first step is to find medical and health care professionals
who are knowledgeable about Sjögren's syndrome, or willing to
learn, and with whom you are comfortable. Second, you need to
know about medications available by prescription and about over-
the-counter products that might help. If you have other disorders in
addition to Sjögren's, you will want to consider the impact on each
disorder and on your Sjögren's. Finally, medical professionals and
other Sjögren's patients can be important sources for helpful hints.
Just remember: no two patients are alike, and always check with
your doctor to make sure products are safe for you!

Finding the Right Doctor

Regardless of who makes the diagnosis of Sjögren's syndrome, it is a good idea to have a medical doctor coordinate your care. Usually this is a rheumatologist. Some patients rely on a clinical immunologist, family physician, or general practitioner. Your rheumatologist or other primary physician might want to see you only once or twice a year if you have had no problems for a sufficient stretch of time, or he or she might want to schedule you for visits every one to four months, depending on your symptoms and medications.

Because Sjögren's syndrome can affect any part of your body and be exacerbated by other common illnesses, patients often ask if they should use their rheumatologist for everything or if they should see an internist too. This question should be discussed with your doctor. Some rheumatologists feel comfortable handling all aspects of your health and taking the time to do so; they will refer you to a specialist when needed. Others prefer that you call an internist for problems not directly related to Sjögren's.

You should see a dentist and ophthalmologist regularly, whether you suffer severe symptoms or not. Prevention and recognition of problems *before* they become severe are key. A good rule of thumb is to see your dentist three times a year and ophthalmologist twice a year, unless you are on medications that need more frequent monitoring or you are having problems that require more frequent attention.

You will see other specialists depending on your symptoms and which organs and body systems are involved.

Unfortunately, the number of rheumatologists is declining (Hahn 2000). This is bad news for those with Sjögren's syndrome and related diseases. In addition, managed care programs might not have a rheumatologist on staff at all, and it can be difficult to get necessary referrals to see specialists needed to treat Sjögren's syndrome.

While the Sjögren's Syndrome Foundation does not recommend specific physicians, the foundation can provide you with names of medical professionals for your area that other patients have found helpful. Foundation volunteer contacts are available for you to call in your area, and they might help you find a medical center or physician close by.

If you cannot find someone locally with whom you feel comfortable, or if you have developed complications and believe you need additional opinions or help, you might want to look for a specialist at a university or other major medical center that sees many Sjögren's patients. A list of treatment centers can be found on the Sjögren's Syndrome Foundation Web site. This and other resources are discussed at the end of this book.

Medications and Products

No prescription medications existed specifically for Sjögren's syndrome until recently. The first drugs ever to target Sjögren's began to emerge over the last few years along with breakthrough medications for related disorders, such as rheumatoid arthritis and multiple sclerosis. There are also promising avenues of research under exploration today, so we urge you to take a look at chapter 12 for a glimpse at the research currently in progress and the possibilities that this research is generating. In the meantime, we suggest you watch for news of treatment breakthroughs from the Sjögren's Syndrome Foundation and other resources provided at the end of this book.

Before we take a look at specific medications and products, we want to offer some words of caution and advice. First, citing any group of medications or common brand names does not imply endorsement on the publisher's or our part. Second, we advise that you *always* check with your doctor about use of any medication or product.

Those with Sjögren's syndrome and other autoimmune diseases can be extrasensitive to medications and tend to have more side effects and drug reactions than the normal population. According to European studies, 18 percent of Sjögren's patients were allergic to penicillin and 15 percent to sulfur compounds (Jonsson, Haga, and Gordon 2001).

Always tell your doctor about all medications you are taking; any vitamins, herbs, or natural remedies you are using (these might interfere *with* or enhance effects of other medications); and any side effects you experience.

Finally, while we list some of the most commonly reported side effects, these lists are not meant to be comprehensive.

Help for Dry Mouth

Two prescription drugs to treat dry mouth have recently been approved by the Food and Drug Administration. These are Salagen (pilocarpine hydrocholoride) and Evoxac (cevimeline). Both increase saliva production; if one does not work for you or you experience uncomfortable or intolerable side effects with one, try the other. The most common side effect of both drugs is increased sweating, and some patients find that one or both of these drugs increase tear production as well.

Use of a prescription fluoride gel will help protect your teeth from cavities. Your dentist can make custom-fitted trays for your teeth, and you should apply a thin ribbon of fluoride in each tray and place on your teeth for approximately two to five minutes every night before going to bed. Do not rinse your mouth after applying fluoride. Brush-on fluorides are also available. Watch out for fluoride mouth rinses that contain alcohol, which is drying and irritating to the oral tissues.

To fight oral candida, or yeast infections, drugs such as Nystatin are available. A catch-22 exists with this condition, because most prescription lozenges for oral use contain sugar, and sugar increases yeast growth. Formulas made without sugar are available, but their terrible taste makes them intolerable for many potential users.

There are also many nonprescription products for dry mouth, including artificial salivas and mouth coats. Contact the Sjögren's Syndrome Foundation for its up-to-date product list.

Other Things You Can Do

Humidify your bedroom or house. Carry water. Chew sugar-free gum. Beware of sugarless gum; this label means less sugar, not zero sugar. Use lip coats to protect lips and the corners of the mouth from chapping.

Dental Implants

If you are diagnosed and treated for dry mouth early in the course of your disease, you should not lose your teeth. However, diagnosis and treatment can come too late, and losing your teeth can be an unfortunate consequence. Dentures have long been the only solution, and they often don't work well in a dry mouth. Now, oral surgeons are turning to dental implants with greater frequency and success, and while they are expensive and labor-intensive for both doctor and patient, the procedure offers an important alternative and holds promise for improvement in the future.

Treatment of Dry Eyes

Lacriserts, available by prescription and made by Merck, have actually been on the market for a long time. Lacriserts are small rice-grain-size pellets that are placed under the lower lid, between the lid and the eyeball, and release moisture for hours. People with Sjögren's either love them or hate them. Periodic shortages have plagued devoted users.

Several prescriptions are currently under investigation as of this writing. Cyclosporin A is undergoing final testing, and scientists are researching other potential treatments, such as topical androgens and tear-volume-enhancing compounds (Meisler 2001).

Over-the-Counter Products

Moisture drops are the first line of defense for dry eyes. If you use them more than four times a day, you need to be sure they are preservative-free drops. Preservatives found in many eye drops can cause a toxic reaction with too frequent use.

Try drops from different manufacturers until you find one you like. Put in drops before you're conscious your eyes are dry. Your eyes will feel better and avoid the potential complications of dryness when they are kept moist.

If drops don't increase your comfort level enough, ointments are available. Apply a rice-grain-size ribbon to the inside of the lower lid. Ointment can cause blurriness of vision for a while after application, so some people use it just at night. Moisture drops can be used in combination with the ointment. Again, preservative-free is best for ointments. If you cannot tolerate the lanolin found in some preservative-free ointments try switching to another brand. Topical gel-like products are also available. They are more viscous than drops but less so than ointments. They don't tend to blur the vision as much.

Special Procedures

Tear loss is diminished when the ducts through which tears escape are closed. Closing these ducts is called punctal occlusion. Your ophthalmologist can close them in one of two ways: by inserting removable punctal plugs made of silicone (or sometimes, collagen) or by cauterization or laser, a more permanent solution. In the former, plugs have been known to fall out, in which case new ones must be reinserted. In the latter, ducts can infrequently and spontaneously reopen on their own. Your ophthalmologist will probably treat the lower ducts initially to see if their closure improves your symptoms or decreases your need for artificial tears. The upper ducts can be done as well if you need additional retention of tears.

Other Things You Can Do

A tolerably hot, wet washcloth applied over your eyes while they are closed can help ease pain. Eyelid cleansers that clear mucus and debris away can help when blepharitis, a condition that can accompany dry eyes, occurs. Special glasses with side shields (moisture chamber glasses) or goggles can be made to slow evaporation and protect your eyes from the drying effect of wind. The Sjögren's Syndrome Foundation has a list with more information on how to obtain products.

General Medications

Medications that reduce inflammation are frequently used in Sjögren's syndrome and other inflammatory conditions. The Arthritis Foundation publishes a drug guide for arthritis-related conditions every year. Check it out for the most up-to-date information. Those most frequently used for Sjögren's syndrome follow.

NonSteroidal Anti-Inflammatory Drugs (NSAIDs)

NSAIDs (pronounced IN-sayds) reduce inflammation and ease pain. The best known NSAID and often the first line of defense for arthritis-related diseases is aspirin. Aspirin is a natural anti-inflammatory, and it can help keep inflammation and pain under control.

Aspirin is a blood thinner that acts by stopping platelets from sticking together, so if you're prone to blood clots with your Sjögren's syndrome, your doctor might have another reason to put you on aspirin. However, if you're already on another blood-thinning drug, your doctor will probably put you on an anti-inflammatory medication other than aspirin. Some people have stomach upset with aspirin. If you are subject to stomach ulcers or bleeding, you probably should not take aspirin. Any NSAID can cause stomach upset, including stomach and gastrointestinal bleeding, and should always be taken with food or milk (unless you are taking an enteric-coated pill).

If you cannot tolerate aspirin, your doctor might suggest trying one of the many nonaspirin NSAID drugs. Examples of common brand names include Naprosyn, Aleve, Motrin, Tolectin, Relafen, Feldene, and Ansaid. Some are available by prescription only.

NSAIDs work by inhibiting the enzymes necessary to produce prostaglandins, which can cause inflammation and pain. Overdoses can be toxic to the liver and long-term use can affect the kidneys. Consult your doctor if you want to increase your regular dose, such as taking additional aspirin for a headache, or if you want to use more than one kind of NSAID.

Don't confuse acetaminophen with aspirin or NSAIDs, such as ibuprofen. Acetaminophen is a pain reliever and does not greatly reduce inflammation.

Cox-2 Inhibitors

A new category of drugs combats inflammation and is easier on the stomach than either aspirin or other NSAIDs. Examples include Celebrex, Vioxx, and Bextra. Cox-2 inhibitors block the Cox-2 enzyme, impeding production of prostaglandins which cause inflammation. The new Cox-2 inhibitors do not act in the stomach but rather in areas responsible for inflammation.

Corticosteroids (Steroids)

Corticosteroids have been around for a long time. They are powerful drugs, and if a person is experiencing debilitating symptoms or dangerous complications, these drugs can often help resolve them. Prednisone is the most widely prescribed steroid. If you are having a major flare-up, sometimes a short-term dose of prednisone is needed. However, this class of medications comes with potential major side effects associated with long-term use and frequency of use. Corticosteroids can reduce resistance to infection, cause bone loss and osteoporosis, lead to the development of cataracts, cause thinning of the skin, and result in increased appetite, and weight gain, and water retention (the so-called "moon face" is a common side effect). They can also lead to the onset of diabetes.

Disease-Modifying AntiRheumatic Drugs

The drugs we've mentioned so far either suppress the immune system or reduce inflammation or both. Disease-modifying anti-rheumatic drugs are anti-inflammatory drugs that go a step further by actually altering the course of a disease.

Antimalarial Drugs

Antimalarial drugs were developed to fight malaria, but clinicians discovered that these drugs help in some autoimmune diseases, including Sjögren's syndrome.

The most common antimalarial drug prescribed for Sjögren's syndrome goes by the brand name of Plaquenil (chemical name: hydroxychloroquine). Many people with Sjögren's feel much better on Plaquenil and often experience improvement in fatigue, joint and muscle pain, and many other systemic symptoms. If you are prone to blood clots and have antiphospholipid syndrome, antimalarials can help.

If you are on hydroxychloroquine, you must see an ophthalmologist every six to twelve months. Though extremely rare, high doses of antimalarial drugs have been known to cause retinal damage. The chemical makeup of Plaquenil and low dosage prescribed for autoimmune disease reduce this risk. Check with your doctor about other potential side effects and monitoring requirements.

Methotrexate

Methotrexate reduces inflammation. It was developed for certain cancer patients and later found to be helpful for rheumatoid arthritis. Approved for use in rheumatoid arthritis by the Food and Drug Administration in 1988, the drug has been successfully used by many rheumatoid arthritis patients and those with related, overlapping disorders.

This drug is generally reserved for progressive and active, severe disease. Side effects can include reduced ability to fight infection, reduced fertility while on the medication, gastrointestinal symptoms, mouth sores, and shortage of folic acid. Some reports suggest that use of methotrexate can increase the risk of malignant non-Hodgkin's lymphoma. Consult your doctor and your pharmacist for a full list of potential side effects.

Cytoxan or Cyclophosphamide

This powerful immunosuppressant can have a lifesaving impact on *severe* disease. As with other powerful medications, however, benefits need to be weighed against potential risks, since this medication can reduce your ability to fight off infection.

What about Biologic Response Modifiers?

You might have heard about some of these drugs, commonly used for related autoimmune disorders. This class of drugs is relatively new on the market, and testing and research on most of these drugs have been directed towards rheumatoid arthritis. This group includes etanercept (Enbrel), infliximab (Remicade), and the newest—anakinra (Kineret). These drugs reduce inflammation caused by cytokines by blocking TNF-alpha, or tumor necrosis factor- alpha. TNF-alpha is involved in Sjögren's, and the Sjögren's Syndrome Clinic at the National Institutes of Health is investigating the effect of etanercept on Sjögren's. One recent study examined infliximab use in primary Sjögren's syndrome patients and found significant improvement in clinical features, including dry eyes and dry mouth (Steinfeld et al. 2001). Another recent study showed potential negative effects on the nervous system and exacerbation of multiple sclerosis when anti-TNF-alpha therapy was used (Mohan et al. 2001).

Other Specific Symptoms

Because Sjögren's syndrome can affect any body organ or system, patients will face an array of symptoms and potential medications to ease those symptoms. These include:

Reflux. Many prescription and over-the-counter products are available for gastrointestinal symptoms such as reflux. Acid blockers include recognizable brand names such as Tagamet, Zantac, and Pepcid. Over-the-counter varieties can help reflux but are usually insufficient to counteract gastrointestinal effects of NSAIDs. Another category of medication that reduces acid production is the proton-pump inhibitor such as Nexium, formerly named Prilosec, and the commonly prescribed drug Prevacid. Before turning to medication, try elevating the head of your bed by placing blocks of wood under the legs at the head. This alone just might do the trick!

Nerve pain. If you suffer from nerve pain or severe numbness, treating your Sjögren's with one of the systemic medications might help. Prednisone reduces nerve inflammation and might give relief. Gabapentin (Neurontin) is sometimes used by Sjögren's patients for nerve pain, although it was originally designed to prevent seizures.

Antiphospholipid antibody syndrome. If you have this syndrome, you need a blood thinner, or anticoagulant, to prevent blood clots. Your doctor might recommend that you take one baby aspirin a day, or you might need a prescription medication such as warfarin (the brand name you might be familiar with is Coumadin) or heparin.

Autoimmune hearing loss. Patients with autoimmune hearing loss have responded well to corticosteroids and cyclophosphamide. Controlling the autoimmune disease process with anti-inflammatory drugs can be helpful. Diazepam (Brand names Valium and Diastat) has been used in some cases to calm the inner ear in Ménière's disease.

Osteoporosis. If you have been on long-term or high doses of prednisone (or have a family history of osteoporosis), you will want to talk to your doctor about the many drugs available to help prevent osteoporosis. There are new drugs now that not only prevent bone loss but actually build bone. These include Fosamax and Actonel, which are now available in once weekly doses. You may also need to take calcium and vitamin D supplements.

Dryness everywhere! Nasal sprays are available for dry nasal passages. In addition, some people use a nasal irrigator, a device that attaches by a hose to a unit such as the WaterPik, and forces water (or saline or anti-mucus solution) through the nasal passages. Keep your head down over a sink, breathing through your mouth. Place the irrigator in one nostril, let the water flow through one nostril and out the other, and then switch to the other nostril and do the same thing.

Vitamin E capsules can be broken open (the cheapest way to obtain vitamin E oil) and the oil applied to the external area around the vagina. During peri- and postmenopause, your doctor might recommend vaginal suppositories (such as Vagifem), especially if you do not take hormone replacement therapy. Many lubricants are on the market to help dry skin. Again, refer to the product lists distributed by the Sjögren's Syndrome Foundation.

Infections. Because the immune system is not functioning normally in autoimmune diseases, many of us find we are more vulnerable to infections and take longer to fight them off. Prompt recognition and treatment of an infection is important in the Sjögren's syndrome patient to succeed in more quickly combating the infection and preventing complications. For example, eye infections need prompt attention; oral yeast infections can become recurrent and hard to control if not treated immediately; and respiratory infections can lead to bronchitis and pneumonia.

Fatigue. We wish we could tell you there is a magic bullet that will zap your fatigue with Sjögren's syndrome, but the best advice we can give is to tell you to work with your physician to keep your disease activity under control as much as possible. Many medications that control Sjögren's symptoms can help increase your energy levels. The antimalarials and Cox-2 inhibitors often help reduce fatigue and are preferable for long-term use over corticosteroids. In addition to medication, your fatigue can be handled through lifestyle management, including exercise and pacing of activities, as we will discuss later.

Pain. Treatment of pain depends on the cause. If the cause is your Sjögren's, then treating the underlying disease will often help, just as it will help with fatigue. If you are experiencing muscle and joint pain, then the same anti-inflammatories that help the disease will be your first line of defense. If your mouth pain is caused by a yeast infection, you need to treat that infection. For nerve pain, your options include trying medications that treat your Sjögren's in general or specific drugs targeted to the nerves. When standard therapies are not working, some people turn to natural remedies to help them deal with fatigue and pain—a topic we turn to next.

Natural Remedies

Many people will tell you they heard about a remedy that could be a sure or potential cure for your Sjögren's syndrome. We are certainly open to the possibility that some of those remedies might prove beneficial in the long run, but until they are: Beware! Just because something is natural, this does not make it safe or appropriate. Aspirin is "natural," but it can have undesirable side effects as well as benefits. Other natural remedies can be quite powerful, and you should watch out for potential interactions with other medications you're taking.

Science is all about investigating old and new ideas and learning by testing hypotheses. If you want to use a remedy that is not approved for use in Sjögren's or is not widely embraced by the medical community, talk to your doctor about it. Some vitamins and supplements have been proven to be helpful in Sjögren's. Vitamin C is a natural anti-inflammatory, but too much can cause stomach upset, diarrhea, and kidney problems. Vitamin B_6 can help inflamed nerves, but again, too much can be detrimental.

Therapeutic massage is safe, and we're learning more about its therapeutic effects. The power of positive touch can be healing. Acupuncture treatments have also helped some people with Sjögren's syndrome and are gaining in popularity for many conditions. However, no clear evidence links acupuncture to benefits for Sjögren's syndrome.

The National Center for Alternative and Complementary Medicine at the National Institutes of Health is a good source of information on natural remedies.

When You Have More Than One Disorder

Sometimes, treatment for one disorder can impact another. Once again, talking over all of your symptoms and treatments with your doctor is critical. For example, many medications effective for allergies or colds cause dryness. If you have Sjögren's syndrome, it's important to know this and to discuss potential alternatives with your doctor. Antidepressants can cause dryness as well.

Because manifestations of Sjögren's syndrome can differ from person to person, a drug that works for someone else with Sjögren's might not be right for you. We have mentioned that the new anti-TNF-alpha drugs might be beneficial for some Sjögren's patients, but if you suffer from neurological difficulties, you and your physician will want to be aware of a potential negative impact on the nervous system. NSAIDs are helpful for many people with Sjögren's but not necessarily for those with a propensity for gastrointestinal side effects.

4

More about the
Medical Aspects

Now that we've discussed the definition, diagnosis, and treatment of Sjögren's syndrome, we know that you will still have specific questions about your individual symptoms and the way Sjögren's affects you. This book is not meant to be a medical textbook with in-depth information about every possible aspect of Sjögren's, but we do want to provide explanations of certain potential symptoms and complications in greater detail.

Your Body and Sjögren's

In this chapter, we examine how Sjögren's can affect different parts of your body. We've organized the chapter so that you can scan it for the topics that especially interest you. Dry eyes and dry mouth are well covered in previous chapters, so we have gone into less detail here. At the end of the chapter, we discuss lymphoma, a cancer that approximately 5 percent of Sjögren's patients develop (Talal 1998).

Your Eyes

Decreased tear production *plus* changes in tear quality contribute to eye symptoms in Sjögren's syndrome. Three layers of tear film—aqueous, lipid, and mucin—make up the eye surface, and each one of them is affected in Sjögren's.

Tearing decreases with age, which is why anyone without dry-eye disease can occasionally have eye discomfort. It is not normal, however, to develop a dry-eye state with persistent or frequent symptoms (Lemp 1999). We have already mentioned that many common medications can exacerbate dryness, but recently, investigators discovered that if you take hormones for menopause, your risk of dry eyes increases (Meisler 2001), although some women report just the opposite. If you are a woman who is older and taking hormone replacement therapy, your risk of dry eye is likely to be higher. According to a 2000 study at Schepens Eye Research Institute, 70 percent of women taking estrogen alone and 30 percent taking estrogen together with progesterone developed dry eyes (Schaumberg 2001). Low levels of the hormone androgen also contribute to dry eyes, and women have lower levels of androgen than men.

Your Mouth

We don't often think about the joy of spit until we lose the ability to produce it. Unlike tears, saliva production does not naturally decrease because of age. Loss of saliva in Sjögren's affects not only the mouth, as we've already discussed, but other areas of the body as well.

Your Salivary Glands

The major salivary glands are known as the parotid glands (the glands that begin under the ear and extend down the jaw and are commonly known as the "mump glands"). These glands are enlarged in one-third to one-half of people with Sjögren's syndrome, changing the lines of your face and creating a slight chipmunklike appearance. The submandibular salivary glands, which lie under the jaw, can also become inflamed and swollen.

Swollen glands can be tender and painful, although not always. Acute pain sometimes signals infections which should be treated.

Recurrent swelling is not uncommon, but your doctor might want to check you for underlying complications if you have had prolonged swelling. Massive enlargement or hard, nodular glands can indicate onset of lymphoma and should be checked.

Your Ears

Dryness can cause itching in the ears. It can also affect the mucous glands of the eustachian tube, resulting in a feeling of stuffiness, muffled hearing, and middle ear infection.

Another potential for ear involvement in Sjögren's is hearing loss. One recent study found 22.5 percent of Sjögren's patients suffered from sensorineural hearing loss of cochlear origin (Politi 2000). Autoimmune inner ear disease with resulting hearing loss can be considered an autoimmune disorder on its own, or it can accompany other autoimmune diseases such as Sjögren's.

Tinnitus and potential hearing loss can be a side effect of certain medications. Aspirin can cause tinnitus, and hearing loss can be a rare side effect of the antimalarial drugs. If a new symptom appears while you are taking any drug, check the list of side effects and consult your doctor.

Your Nose

Dryness of the nasal and sinus passages can cause stuffiness and result in dry crusting and nosebleeds. The nerves and lining of the nasal passages can be damaged, reducing your sense of smell. This, in turn, can affect the taste of food.

Your Throat

The lack of saliva and the effect of Sjögren's syndrome on the mucous membranes impact the throat, creating pain, complicating eating and digestion, and interfering with the vocal cords. Dryness can cause difficulty swallowing, and this can be complicated by lack of motility of the esophagus, atrophy of the mucous lining, and development of abnormal fibrous tissue in the throat. A dry larynx does not function as well as one that is moist, and dryness can make you hoarse. The continuous, dry cough common in Sjögren's, or the need to cough up mucus from the throat, can contribute to sore throat and voice difficulties. Talking dries your mouth and throat further, making public speaking or talking for long periods on the telephone difficult.

Your Digestive System

Saliva aids digestion. From the moment food enters the mouth, the digestive process begins. Those with Sjögren's syndrome are in trouble right from the start!

Mucous membranes that line the mouth and throat extend to the stomach and intestines. Atrophy and potential ulceration of these membranes complicates digestion, successful use of medications, absorption of nutrients, and the ability to fight infection.

Reflux, a common complication of Sjögren's syndrome, contributes to irritation and damage of the esophagus.

Your Pancreas

Sjögren's syndrome can affect the production of digestive enzymes by the pancreas, further complicating digestion. The pancreas can also become inflamed in Sjögren's, a condition called pancreatitis, although this is unusual. Pancreatitis is marked by abdominal pain and increased levels of amylase, a pancreatic enzyme, but because this enzyme is often elevated in someone with Sjögren's, you will need to distinguish whether the increased amylase is of pancreatic or salivary gland origin.

Your Liver

Researchers report frequent abnormal liver findings (liver function or enlargement) in Sjögren's patients, although researchers' percentages vary widely from 25 percent to 58 percent (Fox 1992). If you have abnormal findings, this does not always mean you have liver disease, but it shows once again how Sjögren's can frequently affect many organs. Two autoimmune liver diseases are associated with Sjögren's, primary biliary cirrhosis and autoimmune hepatitis.

Primary Biliary Cirrhosis

Primary biliary cirrhosis (PBC) is the liver condition most closely connected with Sjögren's. About 70 percent of those with this autoimmune liver condition have symptoms of Sjögren's syndrome

(Eskrels 1998), and about 10 percent of those with Sjögren's have PBC (Jonsson, Haga, and Gordon 2001). The main symptoms are itching all over your body and fatigue. PBC causes progressive liver damage and can remain mild or lead to liver failure.

Autoimmune Hepatitis

Autoimmune hepatitis means inflammation of the liver, and inflammation is caused by autoantibodies. The condition can be treated with corticosteroids. Untreated autoimmune hepatitis can lead to cirrhosis, or hardening of the liver, and liver damage.

Your Thyroid

Autoimmune thyroid conditions are commonly found in those with Sjögren's or in family members of someone with Sjögren's. Almost 30 percent of Sjögren's patients have thyroid gland dysfunction or thyroid antibodies (Jonsson, Haga, and Gordon 2001). The thyroid, a small gland just below your Adam's apple, regulates your metabolism. It does this by producing thyroid hormones. In autoimmune disease, specific autoantibodies can cause your thyroid to either overproduce (resulting in Graves' disease) or underproduce (resulting in Hashimoto's thyroiditis) these hormones.

Many of the symptoms of autoimmune thyroid conditions can be confused with symptoms you might already be experiencing from Sjögren's. A simple blood test for hormone levels will provide you and your physician with a quick answer. Your doctor might also test for thyroid antibodies.

Graves' Disease

If you have Graves' disease, your thyroid is hyperactive, meaning you produce too much thyroid hormone. Graves' is known for sometimes causing a bug-eyed look, where your eyes seem to protrude. Your eyes can become inflamed and surrounding tissue swollen. Other signs can include weight loss, a hot and flushed appearance, fast or irregular pulse, muscle weakness, and lighter and less frequent menstrual periods. Graves' can also cause nervousness, irritability, hair loss, and dry hair and nails. Thyroid hormone levels will need to be checked every year because they can change and medication might need to be adjusted.

Hashimoto's Thyroiditis

If you have Hashimoto's thyroiditis, your thyroid tends to be *underactive*, meaning you produce too little thyroid hormone. An underactive thyroid can cause you to gain weight; feel cold, sluggish, and depressed; develop a slow heart rate, muscle cramps, dry and brittle hair, and itchy skin; and have heavier menstrual periods.

Your Lungs

Dryness of the lungs and upper respiratory tract and inflammation of the bronchial glands can lead to bronchitis and recurrent pneumonia. A dry cough is common. You can have difficulty breathing and pain with breathing. Fibrosis, or scarring, of the lung can occur, leading to interstitial pulmonary fibrosis. White blood cells, or lymphocytes, might invade the lung tissue just as they might invade any organ or tissue in the body in autoimmune disease. This lymphocytic infiltration can lead to development of malignant lymphoma, which can sometimes occur in the lungs in those with Sjögren's (accounting for about 20 percent of the lymphomas in Sjögren's) (Hansen 1989).

Your Joints and Muscles

Joint and muscle pains are common symptoms of rheumatic diseases, and Sjögren's syndrome is no exception. Symptoms can include stiffness and pain, especially in the morning.

Your Nervous System

Involvement of your peripheral nervous system (PNS)—that is, the nerves throughout your body excluding the brain and the spinal cord—is not uncommon in Sjögren's syndrome. Antibodies can attack the nerves or blood vessels causing inflammation, and when blood flow to the nerves is impaired, nerve damage can result. For most Sjögren's patients who experience nervous system involvement, the condition is mild and not debilitating.

Your Peripheral Nervous System

Involvement of the PNS usually causes abnormal sensations and primarily affects your legs and feet, and less frequently, your hands and arms. This sensory nerve involvement can lead to decreased sensation, sometimes referred to as a "stocking and glove" sensation and described as tingling, burning, and feeling like pins and needles. You also might have severe pain.

PNS involvement can also affect the cranial nerves, which can become inflamed and cause tingling in the scalp and head and headache, and affect your sense of taste and smell and even your eyesight. A condition called trigeminal neuralgia, the most common cranial nerve involvement, can cause facial numbness and pain and even make the surface of your eyeballs numb.

Another common type of PNS involvement is entrapment neuropathy, in which a nerve becomes numb because it's "trapped" or compressed. Carpal tunnel syndrome is a common example. In this syndrome, the wrist and hand become numb when the median nerve is compressed, or trapped by swollen tissue. Another example is tarsal tunnel syndrome, which causes burning and pain in the bottoms of your feet when walking or cycling.

Motor nerves are infrequently involved, but when they are involved, motor activities, including walking, balance, and manual dexterity can be affected.

The autonomic nervous system is part of your peripheral nervous system and includes nerves controlling involuntary or semivoluntary nerve actions. Involvement of the autonomic nervous system can cause decreased sweating, affect your ability to regulate body temperature, contribute to decreased tears and saliva and difficulty swallowing, cause dizziness, and involve the bowel and bladder and result in incontinence.

Peripheral nerve involvement is often marked by periodic and spontaneous improvement, so unless the pain or numbness is extreme, further testing or treatment probably will not be offered. Electrophysiologic studies (such as electromyography and nerve conduction tests) can determine the extent of damage to peripheral nerves, but these tests will only pick up on major damage. Most people with peripheral neuropathy test positive for the autoantibody SSA.

Your Central Nervous System

The brain and spinal cord make up the central nervous system (CNS). CNS involvement in Sjögren's syndrome clearly occurs in some patients (Pillemer 2002), although the extent of the problem in Sjögren's remains controversial. While CNS involvement in lupus became well-established long before that in Sjögren's syndrome, a group at Johns Hopkins finally brought the Sjögren's-CNS connection to the fore in the 1980s, and studies continue to emerge in this interesting area.

CNS involvement in Sjögren's can resemble multiple sclerosis, and your neurological symptoms in Sjögren's can mimic or be misdiagnosed as multiple sclerosis. You might develop cognitive dysfunction, including problems with memory and concentration.

If your doctor suspects CNS involvement, he or she will probably order a brain MRI, which can show evidence of white matter—or spots of signal intensity—and perhaps test your spinal fluid. Many other tests that provide greater information about the brain and spinal cord, such as electrophysiologic studies, cerebrospinal fluid analysis, and cerebral angiography, might only be offered at major medical centers. Until you experience multiple or severe and damaging events of CNS, treatment is often conservative and physicians prefer to keep a close watch. If you do need treatment, powerful immunosuppressive therapy, administered intravenously and usually by a method called pulse therapy (given intermittently), is successful and problems can even be reversed (Alexander 1998). The immunosuppressives of choice in this case are corticosteroids or cyclophosphamide.

Your Vascular System

The nervous and vascular systems are closely interrelated, so if you have neuropathy (a disease of the nerves), you might also have vasculitis, which is inflammation of your blood vessels. Vasculitis in Sjögren's syndrome is usually restricted to the small blood vessels, where immune complexes and antibodies cause inflammation and destruction. This process can impact many organs, because if blood flow does not reach tissues, the tissue can be damaged and organ function affected. If medium-size arteries are affected, blood flow to the fingers and toes can be reduced, leading to tissue death, or gangrene.

Capillaries that are destroyed can cause blood to leak just under the skin. This can show up as reddish purple spots, or purpura. Small hemorrhaging can lead to small red spots called petechiae.

Antiphospholipid Antibody Syndrome

In antiphospholipid antibody syndrome (APLS), autoantibodies to phospholipids (a type of fat) increase your risk of blood clots. If you have APLS, you are at increased risk for deep vein thrombosis, stroke, heart attack, and pulmonary embolism (when a blood clot travels to the lungs). APLS can cause miscarriages, so if you're trying to become pregnant, it's important to be tested for this syndrome.

Nearly 5 percent of primary Sjögren's patients and 13 percent of secondary Sjögren's patients have APLS. The syndrome is *not* associated with an increased incidence of central nervous system involvement in Sjögren's (Alexander 1998). However, if you have both APLS and the autoantibody SSA, your chances of developing vascular disease increases.

APLS will be diagnosed if you have both anticardiolipin antibodies and the lupus anticoagulant in conjunction with episodes related to blood clotting, together with problems such as miscarriages, strokes, and heart murmers.

Raynaud's Phenomenon or Disease

Cold can cause blood vessels to constrict, reducing blood flow and turning fingers red, white, and blue. Ulceration can occur. This condition can be called either Raynaud's phenomenon or Raynaud's disease, depending on its severity (see chapter 2). Raynaud's is frequently associated with Sjögren's as well as other autoimmune disorders.

Your Skin

Dry, flaky skin is a common feature of Sjögren's. Dryness leads to itching, which can get worse in the winter with dry air. Scratching can lead to infection.

You might develop hives or rashes. Reaction to sunlight, especially evident in patients positive for the antinuclear antibody SSA, can result in a rash. If you have a butterfly-shaped rash across your nose and cheeks, your doctor will suspect lupus.

The skin's appearance reflects many autoimmune complications. If you have Raynaud's, your fingers change color. In vasculitis, red and purple spots appear, especially on extremities, and autoimmune liver disease causes a yellowish cast to the skin all over your body. If you suffer from scleroderma along with your Sjögren's, you can develop rough, hardened skin and your skin can lose its elasticity.

Your Hair

Hair can be dry, brittle, and dull in Sjögren's. Hair loss can occur with autoimmune diseases, including Sjögren's, a condition known as *alopecia*. Hair loss can also occur in the autoimmune thyroid disorder, Graves' disease.

Your Heart

Heart problems are unusual in Sjögren's syndrome and are more often correlated with lupus. Sjögren's and lupus are closely associated, however, and heart problems can, indeed, occur. Just as inflammation of the lung lining can take place, inflammation can affect the lining of the heart. This condition is called pericarditis. In addition, irregular and slow or fast heart rates can occur with auto-immune thyroid disorders.

Your Kidneys

Just like other organs, the kidneys can become inflamed in Sjögren's syndrome, leading to interstitial nephritis. This type of inflammation makes it difficult to produce concentrated urine, so you urinate more frequently and in greater volume. Renal tubular acidosis can also occur and lead to potassium depletion. A third and rarer kidney complication in Sjögren's is glomerulonephritis, which is more commonly found in lupus.

How do you know you have kidney complications? People often think of lower back pain as being connected with the kidneys, but this symptom is not found in autoimmune kidney disorders. Most likely you would have no symptoms, although you might experience swollen ankles and a feeling of abdominal bloating. Evidence usually starts with abnormal urinary and blood tests. Your urinalysis might show excess protein, called proteinuria; blood urea nitrogen (BUN) and creatinine levels can also point to a potential kidney problem.

Your Bladder

Urinary complaints are not uncommon in Sjögren's syndrome. We all know that drinking liquids throughout the day and night leads to numerous trips to the bathroom and disruption of sleep. Bladder irritation can occur and bladder inflammation sometimes accompanies Sjögren's. Urinary frequency, urgency, and pain can ensue (Haarala et al. 2000).

Your Reproductive System

Moisture production in the vaginal area is frequently depleted in Sjögren's, affecting the health of the vaginal tissues and causing an increased tendency for developing infection and experiencing pain during intercourse.

Planning a pregnancy with Sjogren's syndrome requires some special considerations:

* Are you taking medications that might interfere with your becoming pregnant or that you will have to stop taking if you should become pregnant?

* Do you have an antiphospholipid antibody that could interfere with a pregnancy?

* If you have anti-SSA and/or anti-SSB antibodies, have you talked with your doctor about the possibility of complete heart block (a complication that occurs in babies born to mothers with these antibodies)? In heart block, an abnormally low heart beat is detected between twenty and thirty weeks of gestation. This cardiac problem develops because the normal electrical signals that regulate fetal heartbeat are interrupted by the mother's autoantibodies (Buyon 1998).

Hormone changes in pregnancy can impact the autoimmune disease process in the mother. Sometimes the change is for the better—many women say their Sjögren's syndrome improves during pregnancy. Sometimes the change is for the worse; some women report flare-ups during the roller coaster changes in hormones. You and your doctor will have to determine which medications you can continue during pregnancy and weigh your need for disease control with the potential impact of medications on the fetus.

Is it safe to take hormone replacement therapy for menopause or hormones for birth control? We don't know. Studies have shown contradictory results and this topic continues to be hotly debated. Because estrogen is known to cause flare-ups in autoimmune disease, some doctors recommend avoiding it. Many studies have shown hormone replacement therapy to help prevent osteoporosis and cardiovascular problems, so if you are at risk for these problems, you and your doctor might lean toward using this therapy. Recent studies question these benefits, however. More studies are desperately needed.

What Is Lymphoma?

Lymphoma is a cancer involving the lymphatic system, which is part of the immune system. This system includes a network of thin tubes throughout the body (comparable to blood vessels and the body's circulatory system) that carry infection-fighting cells called lymphocytes. Lymph nodes exist along this network and occur in clusters in the neck, groin, underarms, and stomach. If you've had any infection, you might have felt a lump in one of these locations; it was probably a swollen lymph node. The lymphatic system also consists of the bone marrow, thymus, spleen, and tonsils.

Constant stimulation of the immune system increases the chance that something might go wrong. In addition to chronic immune stimulation in Sjögren's syndrome, Sjögren's is marked by lymphoproliferation and infiltration of moisture-producing glands. This infiltration activity can change from a benign (not malignant) state to one that spins out of control and becomes malignant. Norman Talal, a researcher and clinician in Sjögren's syndrome and also in lymphoma, suggests that while the progression of autoimmune disease to lymphoma does not occur in the majority of cases, it can be termed a natural progression (Talal 1998).

Approximately 5 percent of those with Sjögren's syndrome will develop lymphoma. Scientists have estimated the risk at anywhere between 2 and 10 percent, but most agree with the use of the 5 percent statistic. Compared with the general population, someone with Sjögren's has up to a forty-four-fold increased risk of developing lymphoma.

Non-Hodgkin's Lymphoma

The majority of lymphomas occurring in Sjögren's syndrome are non-Hodgkin's lymphomas. They are also usually low-grade, meaning they develop more slowly and symptoms are less severe than in aggressive lymphomas. The lymphoma process in Sjögren's most often involves the B-cells, white blood cells that are part of the immune system. T-cell lymphomas can also occur but are less frequent.

Sjögren's syndrome largely targets the mucous membranes, and the type of non-Hodgkin's lymphoma correlated with Sjögren's affects these membranes. It's called "mucosa-associated lymphoid tissue" lymphoma, or MALT. This location is where the autoimmune disease process most likely crosses over into a malignant process. The salivary glands are a predominant site for the onset of lymphoma in Sjögren's.

You might hear other terms in your search for information about cancer and Sjögren's syndrome which we'll briefly mention. Multiple myeloma is a cancer of the bone marrow leading to uncontrolled growth of plasma cells (part of the immune system). Leukemia, a cancer of the blood, or white blood cells, is closely related to lymphoma. Finally, B-cell chronic lymphacytic leukemia (B-CLL) can sometimes occur in the autoimmune process.

Scientists have found that specific symptoms and lab results indicate a higher risk of developing lymphoma. This does not mean that everyone with those symptoms and test results will develop lymphoma or is even likely to develop it. What is the percentage of those who do, and of those who don't? We don't know. What is the comparative risk of one high-risk symptom or lab result with another? We don't know. Until long-term studies are done that examine those questions, we will not have that information.

It does not matter how long you have had Sjögren's syndrome. Lymphoma can occur soon after diagnosis or many years later. We should note, however, that the diagnosis of lymphoma prior to a suspicion of Sjögren's is one of the exclusionary factors for definitive diagnosis of Sjögren's syndrome. Does this mean that Sjögren's could not exist earlier? No. It means that Sjögren's was not diagnosed before the lymphoma.

When to Be Concerned

A list of symptoms, conditions, and lab tests evident in most Sjögren's syndrome patients diagnosed with lymphoma follows. If you are positive for these, this does not mean you will necessarily develop lymphoma. Many of these symptoms are common in the normal course of Sjögren's.

Your doctor will focus on the combination of symptoms and what happens with lab tests over time. For example, having a positive rheumatoid factor is common in Sjögren's, and this finding simply means you definitely have autoimmune disease and are therefore in the risk pool for lymphoma along with everyone else who has autoimmune disease. This is also true if you are positive for anti-SSA and anti-SSB and have high levels of immunoglobulins. Your doctor will monitor every one of these, because once they are positive, their drop in numbers could indicate onset of lymphoma. Remember that some medications can cause them to drop, as well.

Your physician will want to monitor the following lab findings:

- Rheumatoid Factor: A positive rheumatoid factor is common in autoimmune disease and simply means that by having an autoimmune disease you may have an increased susceptibility to lymphoma.

- Cryoglobulins: Production of these protein complexes circulating in the blood are spurred on by a positive rheumatoid factor. About one-third of those with Sjögren's have cryoglobulins. They are usually mixed with monoclonal IgG immunoglobulins in Sjögren's.

- Anti-SSA (or *Ro*): One of the autoantibodies common in Sjögren's syndrome is anti-SSA. Having anti-SSA increases the likelihood a person will develop certain symptoms that are also increased in those who develop lymphoma. This antibody is correlated with greater disease severity and increased complications, including lymphoma.

- Low hemoglobin or red blood cell counts (anemia).

- Low white blood counts (lymphopenia).

- High ESR, or sed rate.

- Low complement.

* Hypergammaglobulinemia. This term means having a higher than normal number of immunoglobulins, another common feature in Sjögren's.

These clinical signs are associated with increased development of lymphoma:

* Extraglandular disease: Extraglandular means involvement of organs and systems in addition to the moisture-producing, or exocrine, glands.

* Cutaneous vasculitis, or inflammation of the blood vessels visible on the skin.

* Purpura: Bleeding under the skin, causing red and purplish spots similar to bruising and which is a manifestation of cutaneous vasculitis.

* Persistently swollen salivary glands: A recent European study found that 84 percent of those with Sjögren's syndrome who developed lymphoma had bilateral (meaning on both sides of the face) parotid gland swelling (Jonsson, Haga, and Gordon 2001).

* Persistently swollen lymph nodes, or lymphadenopathy.

* Peripheral nervous system involvement.

* Recurring low-grade fever.

Recent reports published in 2001 and 2002 further delineate risks for lymphoma. One study shows that if you were diagnosed at a younger-than-average age with Sjögren's, you will have an increased incidence of swollen lymph nodes and monoclonal immunoglobulins, symptoms which add to your risk of lymphoma (Jonsson, Haga, and Gordon 2001). And, if you had a low complement and palpable purpura (meaning purpura that is raised and can be felt) at diagnosis, your risk for developing lymphoma is higher.

How Lymphoma Develops

Because lymphoma associated with Sjögren's syndrome is usually slow to develop, you might picture its development as part of a continuum; each movement along that continuum places you closer to the potential development of lymphoma. You might also picture yourself as being in a high-risk pool, with your risk increasing with every risk factor you develop. We cannot emphasize enough that possessing these risk factors, however, does not mean you will automatically progress to lymphoma: you might *never* develop further features that predispose you to lymphoma, and you might *never* progress to having a true lymphoma.

You'll frequently hear the term pseudolymphoma in connection with Sjögren's, although lead researchers tell us it is quickly becoming obsolete. This term has been used for years to designate a condition in which lymphocytes accumulate abnormally and you appear to have lymphoma yet do not have a true, lymphoid malignancy. Recent advances in diagnosis are helping doctors to better distinguish whether you actually have malignant lymphoma, making the term pseudolymphoma no longer necessary.

If you have high levels of gamma globulins, or immunoglobulins (IgG, IgM, IgA), that suddenly drop to normal or low numbers, your physician might be concerned with the possibility of lymphoma. The antimalarial drugs can cause your immunoglobulin levels to drop to normal, however, so be aware of this benign cause. Sometimes immunoglobulins are low for years before a person develops lymphoma.

The appearance of a monoclonal spike (also known as an M-spike or myeloma spike) in the immunoglobulins is a development to watch closely. A spike is an abnormal clustering or aggregate of immunoglobulins, and an M-spike is an aggregate of monoclonal immunoglobulins. M-spikes are not rare in Sjögren's. If the M-spike grows or is especially high, your physician might recommend further investigation.

Just as a drop in the level of immunoglobulins is a sign for concern, so is a drop in autoantibodies and rheumatoid factor, once you are positive for these. Your physician will also watch for light chains, monoclonal immunoglobulins or proteins, and other proteins in your electrophoresis test, more clearly seen in urine than in blood. You may also hear about a number of highly sophisticated tests that are not done routinely but which some physicians consider useful in assessing risk of lymphoma, such as the blood test for emergence and increase of beta 2 microglobulin.

Enlarged lymph nodes, and a particularly hard salivary gland or lymph node, will prompt a further look. A hard salivary gland might occur because of a blocked salivary gland or infection. In lymphoma, the node is less movable than when enlarged due to inflammation or infection.

Malignant Lymphoma

Specific signs of concern for malignant lymphoma include chronically swollen and unusually large parotid or lymph glands; fever; weight loss; muscle weakness; significant drop in levels of immunoglobulins, autoantibodies, or rheumatoid factor; development of monoclonal spike; constant fatigue; night sweats not associated with perimenopause; skin rashes; and itching.

Chronically swollen and unusually large parotid glands can be symptomatic of lymphoma. These glands extend from the ears and down along the chin line. "Unusually large" means these glands are huge, each taking up half of one side of your face.

Chronically swollen and unusually large lymph glands that remain swollen for more than a week or continue to grow can be a sign for concern. High fever without an explanation can signal the onset of a malignancy, and it can also occur with neurological complications of Sjögren's. Low-grade fevers can occur in Sjögren's with no evidence of malignancy. Night sweats can indicate lymphoma, but you should not confuse this occurrence with night sweats that normally occur during perimenopause.

Weight loss, muscle weakness, and itchy skin, each of which can have other causes such as autoimmune thyroid disorder, can accompany lymphoma. Dry skin alone can cause the skin to itch. Itching connected with lymphoma is more closely akin to a feeling of having hives. Skin rash can be a common feature of autoimmune diseases and alone does not indicate potential lymphoma.

Other signs of lymphoma, such as constant and extreme fatigue, can easily be confused with common symptoms of autoimmune disease. You can have extreme fatigue with Sjögren's, so you and your doctor will have to determine if the fatigue is unusual in any way and if this new fatigue accompanies any of the other signs of lymphoma.

It's critically important when suspecting lymphoma for you and your doctor to look at your whole medical picture—all your symptoms, blood work, and how you feel. The approach to diagnosis will vary depending on your symptoms. Your physician might choose to take a closer look at your whole lymphatic system using X-ray, CAT scan, or MRI technology. A lymphangiogram, in which a dye is used to outline the lymph vessels and nodes, might be done at the same time. A needle aspirate or biopsy of the lymph node or salivary glands will be done if you have swollen or hard nodes. Biopsies are the most definitive diagnostic tool for lymphoma. Remember, however, that the lymphocytic infiltration that is a normal part of Sjögren's syndrome might make it difficult to distinguish between a benign and malignant process. These tests can help your physician determine how advanced the lymphoma is.

Other Issues

As with any chronic illness, coping with Sjögren's means that you have to make adjustments. These can range from taking special care when undergoing surgery to dealing with daily concerns.

Undergoing Surgery

If you have Sjögren's syndrome and are scheduled for elective surgery, you need to be aware of potential complications. Anesthesia can dry you out, so make sure your surgeon and anesthesiologist know you have Sjögren's, that you will need a mouth and lip coat and eye ointment before surgery, and that they will need to be reapplied during and afterward if the procedure is lengthy. Ask for ice chips and rinse your mouth with water up until the last possible moment. Some commonly used herbs are known to change heart rate and blood pressure, interfere with blood clotting, and intensify the effects of anesthetics and narcotics, so make sure you tell your surgeon and anesthesiologist about all the drugs you are taking, including prescription, herbal, and over-the-counter medications.

Sensitivity to Drugs and the Environment

As we've mentioned, people with Sjögren's syndrome frequently experience increased sensitivity to medications and their environment. Allergic reactions have been documented in 65 percent of those with Sjögren's (Jonsson, Haga, and Gordon 2001). 20 to 25 percent of people with lupus are believed to suffer from allergies and sensitivities to substances compared with 10 percent of the general population (Wallace 1995).

Dealing with Fatigue and Depression

You may feel that when you complain about tremendous fatigue, your friends, family, and physicians look at you as if you are crazy and they can't get rid of you quickly enough. Fatigue is tough to see or measure. But many physicians feel fatigue is very real and is a major cause of debilitation in Sjögren's.

Depression is another one of those symptoms often swept under the rug. We talk more about depression in chapter 7, but for now, it might comfort you to know that many leading physicians recognize that depression is common in Sjögren's.

What You Can Do Now

Sjögren's syndrome can affect any organ in the body and range from merely irritating to debilitating symptoms, from noncritical organ dysfunction to malignancy and life-threatening circumstances. Knowing and understanding all the possibilities can be frightening, but we believe that knowledge can be a powerful tool for maintaining control and oversight of your illness. Knowledge can help lead to early treatment and can actually lower your fear level since imagination and unanswered questions can sometimes be more frightening than accurate knowledge.

Other tools you can use to make your disease more manageable include developing a positive relationship with the medical health professionals who treat you and learning to deal positively with your emotions and reactions to illness. We discuss these tools in the upcoming chapters.

5

Doctors and Patients

When you are sick, your doctor should be your mainstay or lifeline, according to Susan Wells, the author of *A Delicate Balance* (2000), a book about living with an autoimmune disease. She describes her physician in the following words: "My doctor was a lifeline for me. He was my primary care physician, my rheumatologist, and my friend. He uttered those magical words, 'I believe you don't feel well . . .' My doctor read information I brought him, and we laughed together at some of the more frustrating, but funny, aspects of my health problems. . . . He wasn't perfect, and he didn't make me well, but he helped me by empowering me to take care of myself. This is the kind of doctor we all want and are sometimes lucky enough to find."

Choosing the Right Physician

Your physician should be a person who can understand how you feel. A visit to a physician that makes you feel lighter, as if a weight has been lifted or at least shared, is one definition of a successful visit. For a person with an illness, much of what is happening is new, strange, and distressing. An experienced physician brings his or her experience and knowledge into your treatment and moves you towards stability and health.

Since Sjögren's is a chronic disease, the goal of the doctor-patient relationship is to minimize complications and treat new symptoms and problems in the most effective manner. Sometimes the goal is to achieve stability, or to return the individual to a more stable state.

A physician treating a chronic, multisystem disease has much to consider. She or he needs to be able to listen effectively in order to anticipate and treat new developments as soon as they begin and keep track of anything that might be pending. Sjögren's and other chronic autoimmune diseases bring out the physician's capacity as healer. The physician helps heal that which cannot be cured.

The doctor-patient relationship is a relationship between individuals, and the individual personalities of both people play a role in determining whether or not the relationship will work. As in any relationship, there needs to be an empathic bond between patient and physician. They should respect and like each other, and be willing to tolerate each other's idiosyncrasies. Communication is of paramount importance. The patient who fears her doctor's criticism or scorn will hesitate to tell her physician what is on her mind. The physician who does not listen well, who is distracted or inattentive, may miss something important.

What do patients want in a physician? Especially with regard to their primary care physician or rheumatologist, they want someone who is accessible, responds, listens well, can empathize, and is well informed about what is wrong with them. Patients want to know their physician will be there if serious problems arise. They want someone who is compassionate and who can appreciate that we will all, sooner or later, become patients and need help.

Most of the people we spoke with realistically accepted the limitations of human nature, and did not expect their physicians to know everything. They asked that their physician not be callous or indifferent, and not say, as one physician did when he could not be bothered to investigate a patient's problem: "You have a chronic disease. You're bound to feel bad."

Dealing with Doctors

Sjögren's syndrome is a disease that requires considerable immersion in the medical establishment. Since it is a multisystem disease, many different specialists can become involved. Often, it feels like too many. In a 1997 essay appearing in the newsletter of the Sjögren's Syndrome Foundation, Teri wrote: "I spend a lot of time sitting in doctor's offices, waiting for my turn, waiting for a doctor to call, waiting for results of one test or another that might or might not change my life. Recently, while filling out a form, I stopped when I wrote 'psychologist' in the space for occupation. It is what I do, but as a psychologist with a chronic disease, I find myself increasingly occupied with being a patient, my time taken up with the business of being ill. Now, I know why we're called patients. Being sick requires an inordinate amount of patience. . . . I try to be patient with the medical profession's attitude of 'hurry up and wait.' It takes patience to have to put something off because I'm not up to it today, patience when the disease gets in the way of having a life. Sometimes, I get downright impatient with it all" (Rumpf 1997, 5).

Waiting in doctors' offices can become the equivalent of a full-time job, an unwelcome, unwanted, and unappreciated occupation. On the other hand, the knowledge that a supportive physician is close at hand provides comfort, calm, and a sense of impending relief. Especially at the beginning, when it is most common for people to see many different physicians for symptoms that may be seemingly unrelated, the multitude of physicians can be a stressful experience.

Since medical specialties do overlap, it can be difficult to know which physician to turn to. Managed care has dealt with this by making the internist or family practitioner the gatekeeper. Even when an individual's insurance allows a patient to go directly to a specialist, a rheumatologist or internist helps define a specific problem, make an initial diagnosis, and refer to the appropriate specialist.

It is important to have someone coordinate and head the team. It is also helpful when this physician knows (or knows about), the other doctors involved, and is able to communicate with them. Since many networks of physicians now have online connections, accessing information is easy when physicians are in the same group or network. When they are not, it is common practice for consulting physicians to send a note to a primary care doctor, rheumatologist, or both. You can ask for this to be done, or offer to do the coordinating yourself. Many people like to keep copies of their own medical records.

Some physicians have little tolerance for patients with chronic diseases, and, like patients, wish for clear and easy answers. Rheumatologists choose their specialty with the awareness that they are not going to cure most of their patients. They understand that their patients will need lifelong care, and that their job is to help you maximize your health. Rheumatologists are not uniform in their knowledge of Sjögren's syndrome. Some have had relatively little experience with it. If you can, try to find a physician who is knowledgeable, experienced, has had other patients with Sjögren's, and who is willing to continue to learn.

Some rheumatologists have a greater tolerance for ambiguity than others. They understand that Sjögren's is part of a group of diseases that can overlap and that a diagnosis can be difficult to make. Some make rapid diagnostic decisions, while others will delay until they feel certain of what they are dealing with. The physician waits, putting the pieces of the puzzle together until she or he is able to reach a definitive diagnosis. The patient waits too, with less detachment and sometimes with great anxiety, to see what will evolve.

The Diagnostic Process

A diagnosis is not completely objective. Some physicians will read a disease one way, while others may have a different interpretation. Autoimmune diseases are not clear-cut. They have subtleties and nuances that leave room for interpretation and subjectivity. Given all the variables, here are some things about the diagnostic process to consider.

The Initial Encounter

In the beginning, it is important that a doctor takes a thorough history. A history is a way for a physician to learn about your experience of your illness, and to examine you for signs of disease. A good history enables the physician to learn something about you. It is more than just medical facts. The way you tell your story provides information about the way you live and cope with problems. Are you anxious, depressed, hopeful or hopeless, organized or scattered? Do you appear sick, weak, or well? The physician notes these impressions, filing them away for future reference. Over time, patterns will emerge, and physicians who know their patients look for what is out of the ordinary. Does a patient who usually looks well appear sick? Is a patient who is well-groomed suddenly unkempt? Initial impressions form a baseline for the future.

We believe that a good history takes place in the doctor's office, not an examining room. If an examining room is all that is available, the history should be taken with both patient and physician sitting at a desk. Unfortunately, checklists are replacing histories, and initial encounters take place with the patient seated on the examining table in order to save a few minutes of valuable time.

In addition to history taking, the initial appointment is the time for a thorough medical exam. The physician touches the patient and gets a baseline sense of the anomalies of the patient's body. Words and touch were the physician's original tools, and although they have been augmented with sophisticated technology, they are still the most fundamental components of the medical encounter. The nature of the doctor-patient relationship gives the physician permission to touch the patient, and this investigative touch is in the service of a relationship based on healing. The physician probes in order to find out what is wrong, and what is all right.

Another special aspect of the relationship is that it allows for intimate disclosure. A patient may disclose things to a physician that he or she has told no one else, because this is a relationship based on trust. If the patient does not trust the doctor, there will be no relationship (Lown 1996).

A first appointment is usually longer to allow for the history and physical examination. It gives you an opportunity to evaluate whether this is a physician with whom you can work, whether the physician is one you are willing to trust with intimate physical and emotional details. The way in which physicians approach the history and physical reveals a great deal about the way they conduct their practice: how well they listen, how sensitive or empathic they are, how available and attentive they are likely to be. When everything goes well, you should leave feeling that you have found someone with whom a working relationship is possible.

Often, more than a single encounter is necessary before this decision can be made. Sometimes a relationship begins with what appears to be a great rapport, but it collapses when there is a crisis to which the physician does not respond. It is important to find someone who responds well in both routine and emergency situations.

It is also possible to know that a relationship will not work on the basis of a single encounter. For example, a physician who meets you for the first time in the examining room and asks, "Would you please tell your history to the medical student I am working with, who will then relay it to me?" is a good example of someone you might like to avoid.

As you talk with your doctor, you can ask some basic questions that will give you a lot of information about how he or she handles patients. Ask yourself how well the two of you seem to communicate. How do you feel about the way he or she responds to you? Does this doctor seem to understand what you are saying?

Questions to Ask before and during an Initial Appointment

* Where is the office located? Can you get there on your own, or does someone need to accompany or take you there?

* How much does this doctor know about Sjögren's syndrome, lupus, and other autoimmune diseases? Does he or she have other patients with Sjögren's?

* How easy is it to get an appointment with this physician? A routine appointment? A special appointment when there is a problem?

* What is the physician's policy regarding lab results and questions?

* How promptly will she or he respond to phone calls? Is e-mail available?

* What is the doctor's policy about emergencies and after-hours phone calls? What happens on weekends? Does the physician take his own calls or are the calls referred to a

covering physician? If the latter, will this doctor have access to your chart?

- If you need to go to the emergency room, how far away is it?

- If you are hospitalized, will this doctor see you in the hospital, or will someone else be responsible for your care? If so, who will that be?

- How will this doctor coordinate your visits to other specialists?

Follow-Up Visits

The interval between visits should be determined by your doctor and you. You will need to see your doctor to follow up on ongoing or new problems. A visit to your doctor can also provide emotional comfort in dealing with a chronic disease. When the disease is stable, between one and four appointments a year may suffice. When problems arise, additional time is needed.

Since follow-up visits are generally shorter than the initial encounter, we advise making a list of problems with the most troublesome at the top of the list. If there are more than three or four separate issues, it may be necessary to schedule another appointment. Need for discussion time varies.

Going to the doctor takes energy. When you feel depleted, it can be difficult to get up enough energy to keep the appointment. On the other hand, most people approach their doctors' appointments with the hope that something will happen that will make them feel better. A scheduled visit when symptoms are active is opportune. It is easier to describe symptoms when they are ongoing.

It's also important to let your physician see you in both good and bad times, so keep your appointments even when there have been no new developments. You can use these times to ask general questions about the illness or about any concerns that you have that you wouldn't ask when you have more urgent problems.

Getting Second Opinions

You should never feel guilty about wanting a second opinion, especially given the overlap and uncertainty with autoimmune diseases. Your physician should not react defensively to your request, and you need not feel disloyal, either in telling your physician that you would like such a consultation or in asking for lab results and a letter explaining the nature of the disease and its course. The consultant may wish to see previous lab results, so it is best to bring these records with you. He or she may also want to repeat some tests or do additional ones.

A second opinion may corroborate the first physician's findings, or it may add new information. Even when no new information is obtained, a second opinion that corroborates or confirms an initial diagnosis or course of action can help you feel more confident in your treatment.

A second opinion always offers the potential for further confusion of a given issue. When this happens, you have to decide whether to seek a third opinion, live with the conflict, or adopt the opinion that makes the most sense (while keeping the alternative filed away, in case it turns out to be correct).

While some insurance plans allow for second opinions, others are not always willing to pay, so it is best to clarify in advance.

Continuity of care may be of particular importance in autoimmune diseases, since Sjögren's syndrome and related diseases tend to develop over long periods of time. A physician who knows you also knows your style. He or she knows whether you are likely to underreport symptoms or be alarmed by them. Though continuity of care is important, you should change doctors if you have the persistent feeling that you are not being helped. Sometimes finding the right physician is a journey in itself.

Ann's Story

This is a story of one woman's search for a physician she could work with and trust. At the beginning of her illness, Ann was tentatively diagnosed with rheumatoid arthritis by her primary care physician. She did not feel comfortable with the diagnosis, so she asked to see a rheumatologist who worked for her health maintenance organization. She waited three months for the appointment, hoping to find out what was really wrong with her. She carefully organized her notes in preparation. She approached the consultation with a mixture of anticipation and dread.

On the appointed day, her hopes fell flat. The consultant gave her just three minutes of his time. He walked into the room, listened briefly, gave her a cursory physical exam and said, "I agree with everything your internist has said." He turned to leave.

"Wait a minute," Ann managed to say. "What's wrong with me?" The consultant was annoyed. He had already pronounced sentence. "I think you have rheumatoid arthritis," he said, echoing the original diagnosis Ann had been given, "just as your internist told you."

Ann climbed down from the examining table, cried with disappointment, then switched her insurance.

Some months later, she went to a second rheumatologist. This one was very thorough and an independent thinker. He took lots of blood tests and ruled out a variety of other illnesses, which reassured Ann. He did not rule in a specific diagnosis. It was, he said, too early to tell. Ann would have to wait and see what developed, but in the interim, he would monitor her and treat what symptoms she had. "I think you look better than you feel," he said, and Ann began to feel that he had seen this before and understood. She could accept the uncertainty as long as there was someone who would share it with her. She was initially impressed with his years of experience and his technical competence, and relieved by the fact that he didn't rush to make a decision right away but wanted time to consider her situation. His thoroughness and intelligence impressed her. She was sure that this doctor would think about what was wrong with her.

"Don't worry too much about this," he said, "and don't make yourself an invalid too soon. Avoid stress." Ann was a single mother who needed to work. She pushed herself to her limits each day. It was impossible not to worry about a disease that had no name and was changing and threatening her quality of life.

She continued to see this rheumatologist for two years. After each visit, she found herself feeling worse than she had before. She was searching for an empathic connection that did not exist. She began to wonder whether all patients in this doctor's practice were happily married women who did not need to worry about their finances, health insurance, or future security.

The rheumatologist didn't seem to understand Ann's anxiety and depression. One day, Ann attended a lecture on the different patterns of antinuclear antibodies (ANA) and the clinical manifestations that might be expected with each. She mentioned this to her physician several weeks later. "You don't need to concern yourself with things like that," he said. "You probably can't understand them anyway." He was wrong.

If fact, several things were wrong. Unlike the first consultant, this physician was not indifferent and he had been extremely thorough. But he really didn't understand Ann's situation. Ann felt increasingly distressed and frustrated by his lack of understanding, despite the fact that she trusted his physical evaluations of her completely.

Finally, Ann went to see a third doctor. When she left his office after their initial meeting, Ann felt as if a weight had been lifted for the first time after three years of being sick. She still had no diagnosis, but finally there was someone who would help her deal with what was happening to her. The rheumatologist had listened and promised her that if he didn't understand something, he was at least willing to try. Here was the collaboration she had been seeking. Almost two decades after seeing the first doctor, Ann has found that this alliance has made a great deal of difference in her illness. Her doctor is someone she can turn to when she needs help and is someone she can trust. He has been a lifeline for Ann. Both doctor and patient know they have a good working relationship.

As this story illustrates, educating yourself, knowing your needs, and being persistent all contribute to finding a physician or physicians who are right for you. We think that it is good to become as educated as possible, as long as you do not become overwhelmed. Although you may want to know everything right away, there's no rush.

Another lesson from Ann's story is that a physician's words can help or hurt. Dr. Bernard Lown, in his book *The Lost Art of Healing* (1996), emphasizes this distinction. With words, a physician has the power to mitigate pain, remoralize, and empower. He or she also has the power to maim. Lown says, "There is absolutely no justification for assaulting patients with language that cows and disempowers. A patient must never be compelled by fear into difficult choices. If there is to be a partnership in medicine, the senior partner has to be the patient, who must not be deflected from having the decisive word" (77).

Medicine and the Marketplace

One of the realities of managed care is that people are often forced to change their health care providers as their medical insurance changes. Not only does this decrease continuity of care; it makes both patient and physician reluctant to become invested in a relationship that may not be ongoing or long-term. But there is a positive side to the increasingly businesslike approach to health care. We are now consumers of health care, and like consumers in any other situation, we have the right to expect satisfaction from our health care providers. This makes it easier to remove yourself from an unsatisfactory relationship and to find one that is more satisfactory.

Technological changes also have transformed the relationship between doctor and patient. Doctors are remunerated for procedures, not for time spent listening or counseling.

Case Studies

Unlike better-known diseases, a diagnosis of Sjögren's is often the result of an odyssey through the medical system. The following stories provide some sense of what people go through before they hear the word Sjögren's. All of these vignettes are here with the permission of their authors. We wish to thank the individuals involved for sharing their stories with us.

Ginger's Story

[I was] diagnosed in 2000 after almost ten years of going from doctor to doctor, including two rheumatologists who kept saying I didn't have an autoimmune disorder because I was negative ANA. Thank God, I found an internist who immediately thought of Sjögren's syndrome and tested me for the anti-Ro and anti-La antibodies, which I blew off the chart. Sjögren's has greatly affected me in many ways I never dreamed possible, especially the joint pain, dry mouth, and gritty eyes. I also have lupus and take an array of drugs to help alleviate the symptoms. Sadly, I have yet to find anyone outside the medical field who has ever heard of Sjögren's syndrome, let alone who knows what it can do to one's body. I hope that increased awareness will come, so that all who face this chronic illness will find not only relief from their symptoms, but for their future as well.

David's Story

I asked four doctors and three dentists over a seven-year period about my dry mouth and dry eyes and nobody could figure it out. Then I searched on the World Wide Web for "dry eyes and dry mouth" and in ten minutes, found out about Sjögren's syndrome. [I've] come to find out, it's not a rare disease—just a disease that many doctors can't recognize.

Sometimes, the patient makes the diagnosis. Alysanne diagnosed herself with Sjögren's, but her doctor dismissed her symptoms and refused to send her to a specialist. Her son was born with complete congenital heart block as a result of the Sjögren's, but even then, her doctor refused to take her seriously. She was finally diagnosed and treated after suffering with the symptoms for many years.

Our own stories are typical of the medical system. Kathy was thirty-two years old before she was diagnosed with Sjögren's syndrome, sixteen years after she began a search for an explanation for her array of symptoms. The doctor at the university medical center where she was diagnosed retrieved and copied his notes on Sjögren's from medical school to provide her with more information. These notes took up only a quarter of one page.

Teri was initially diagnosed with one dry eye. Her ophthalmologist was adamant that it couldn't possibly be anything to worry about, because only one eye was affected. "If you were older," he said, "this might be something to look into." He dismissed it as a curious idiosyncrasy. Years later, in the context of numerous other symptoms, the one dry eye took on a different meaning and began to make sense.

A lack of familiarity with Sjögren's syndrome can lead to a lack of recognition of other problems, even when your doctor makes the correct diagnosis. Potential complications of Sjögren's might be missed and necessary precautions not taken. For example, a simple respiratory infection can become bronchitis and pneumonia in the presence of a compromised immune system. Since patients often look healthy, unknowing physicians treat them as if they had a disease limited to dry eyes and dry mouth, with few other consequences. If you tend to develop infections, inform your doctor and plan ahead so that you can expedite treatment when the time comes.

Emotions and the Medical Encounter

All too often, a visit to a physician does not allow time for discussion of what illness means and how you feel about it. Doctors remain ignorant about how the illness really affects you, even after years of care. Focus on medical symptoms is necessary but not sufficient, we think, because they are only part of the picture. A chronic illness rearranges life as it is lived. The changes and adaptations required affect you, perhaps as much as the medical problems.

The physician will make notes about the physical changes that occur from one visit to the next, but may ask nothing about emotional changes. You learn to report changes or new developments in a neutral way, and all too often, a kind of conditioning occurs. You learn what to include and what to leave out. Of course, this is not always the case. Physicians and their patients often talk frankly about important concerns and emotional changes. These conversations deepen the relationship. If they do not occur, because the physician is too busy, is too matter-of-fact, or limits his or her practice to questions the patient must answer, both of you are shortchanged. The physician doesn't really know you. You never get to say what is on your mind.

Especially in times of crisis, a physician needs to act as an auxiliary ego. This is a psychiatric term for when a situation is too emotionally charged for someone to think clearly and someone else needs to help out in terms of support and decision making. In life, this happens all the time. When we are distressed, we rely on our spouses, partners, friends, and families for advice and help. When the context is a medical problem, we want to be able to depend on the support and advice of our doctor(s), and, this can make the difference between being able to cope and being overwhelmed.

Physician Styles

Physicians use a number of styles in their interactions with patients. Among these are collaborative, authoritarian, interrogative, formal, informal, and paternalistic. A physician's personality influences the style he or she uses, although the way a physician interacts may change with age and experience. The style a doctor uses influences his or her communication with patients. The physician described earlier by Ann was somewhat authoritarian and perhaps paternalistic: Ann didn't need to worry about her disease, because he would take care of things. He would make the treatment decisions. Some people find this style comforting; they want their physician to tell them what to do. Ann obviously did not. It is important to remember that not everyone needs the same qualities in a physician.

An authoritative style can be a good thing when there is an emergency or an acute condition that needs immediate treatment, says Suzy Szasz, a lupus patient who wrote about her experiences in a book called *Living with It* (1991). However, she feels it is not a good style for someone with a chronic disease, because doctor and patient need to form a collaboration and work together. We all want our physician to be an authority—not to be confused with being authoritarian. We want our physician to understand our disease, to be able to tell us what the numbers on our lab results mean, and we want to be sure that our physician will know the correct thing to do when we are sick. The style a physician uses to communicate with a patient is different from what he or she knows.

A physician who uses an interrogative style is likely to structure the interview with questions. When used by a skilled and thoughtful physician, this style generates a great deal of information, although it may preclude telling the physician things which fall outside the scope of the questions. Teri had one of the best consultations of her life with a physician who asked her questions for over two hours. She felt as if they were putting a very complicated jigsaw puzzle together. When they almost were done, she told him that one of the worst manifestations of Sjögren's for her was the overwhelming fatigue. The physician looked up, surprised. "You're right," he said, "I forgot to ask you about that." Had she not spoken up, one very important piece would have been missing.

A collaborative style is one where the physician listens and then asks questions to clarify and elaborate on what he or she has been told. The physician validates and helps you make sense out of the experiences you have had. While it is the physician who determines treatment, there is the feeling of working together to solve a problem.

Patient Experts

Thanks to the increased availability of information, you can now become an expert on Sjögren's and the way it affects you. You know your own body better than anyone else. With careful reading, you can become as informed as you want to be. This means you can bring your expertise to the table when working with your doctor.

We would be remiss if we did not point out that there is also a great deal of misinformation available. There are abundant myths and rumors and unproven treatments that someone will want you to buy. Even when the information is good, most patients do not have the benefit of their physician's years of training and practice and the perspective gained from seeing and treating hundreds, if not thousands, of patients. Ideally, doctor and patient work together as a team.

Patients may be alert to changes that physicians overlook. For example, a lab test result may be in the normal range but may be a departure from the norm for you. If you know what your baseline is, you can point it out, and your physician may decide to watch this particular lab value or to repeat the test. Physicians have much to keep track of. It helps for you to be as aware as possible of what is normal or abnormal for you.

Good Doctor Stories

To have a chronic illness is to enter the world of doctors' offices, appointment secretaries, endless insurance forms, new patient questionnaires, old magazines, paper johnnies, and generalized indifference to the circumstances that necessitated the appointment—being sick. In such a world, a bit of human kindness goes a long way toward making difficult situations tolerable. Small acts of kindness are appreciated at any time. A personal greeting or a kind word from the receptionist at the beginning of an office visit, or a short conversation with the nurse or phlebotomist who draws blood, makes a visit to a medical office better.

We asked more than seven-hundred people on the Sjögren's syndrome listserv to share their positive experiences with doctors or the medical system. Good doctor stories proved to be more difficult to elicit than their opposite. Perhaps when there is a lack of rapport or an unsatisfactory encounter, the outrage is carried for longer periods of time and people jump at the chance to tell these "bad doctor" stories. We did get a number of responses, however. Here are some of the "good doctor" stories we received.

Janice's Story

I have a terrific internist who has been known to call me in the evenings, from her home, to check on me, after I've been in her office with something major going on. She's very caring, is a terrific listener, and always seems to have a lot of time for me during office visits. When she doesn't know something about my health, she told me that she has, from time to time, contacted one of her old professors at Boston University to talk with him about my situation. I find that very refreshing, that she's willing to help.

Bobette's Story

After eight years of living with a myriad of symptoms and getting no diagnosis or help from anyone, I found the most wonderful doctor anyone could ever have. He gave me a good part of my life back. What sets him apart from other doctors is that he listens, and listens carefully. No complaint is ever dismissed. He will address personal problems that arise from the disease as well as physical. He is a caring physician who has volunteered to be the medical advisor for our support group. He attends our meetings on Saturdays and has helped write a cookbook for people with dry mouth. I believe he can truly empathize with his patients. Now, when any new symptom arises, I know where to turn.

Max's Story

I saw an oral medicine specialist, a specially trained DDS, who is also a researcher into Sjögren's and other causes of dry mouth. What she did for me was to persuade me, Mr. Natural Non-Pill Popper, that it is useful to treat dry mouth aggressively. She scraped a thick coating of candida off my tongue, to make me aware of this problem, and went into some detail explaining things, not holding back on the complexity when she saw I was keeping up with her explanation. It was a pleasure to be treated as though I had some intelligence.

In the second case, I had been unable to strike up a good working relationship with my ophthalmologist. Part of it was the assembly line format. A doctor in training would ask me questions and make notes, then the doctor would treat the notes, not me. . . .

On to the good part. I became aware of another ophthalmologist when she spoke to our local chapter of the Sjögren's Syndrome Foundation. She seemed to be open to trying things and was a good and careful listener. . . . At the end of the appointment I walked out almost dazed from having my ophthalmological frustration changed into a sense of fulfillment. She often runs an hour late, but for me, being included in the discussion, and an active participant in my own treatment, is worth a lot.

With both the oral medicine specialist and the ophthalmologist, I was searching, based on a vague feeling that there might be better help out there than I was getting. Fortunately, I had no insurance-based constraints on my choice of physicians. I was not looking at a time of crisis, but more along the lines of trying to consolidate my position and make steady improvements in my medical team.

Max's final point is one we wish to highlight. While crisis often forces people to seek a second opinion, it is not the best time to make changes in your medical team. A better time is during a period of relative stability, when there are no pressing or emerging problems.

Being a Patient

Sometimes it feels as if living is what takes place in between doctor's appointments. You find yourself stuck within the boundaries of your body, and find that preserving whatever health remains now takes a substantial amount of your time and energy. Even as the medical system breaks you down into dry eyes, dry mouth, and the results of your lab tests, it is important to remember that you are more than the sum of your body parts.

Before the onset of chronic illness, we were able to take our bodies for granted. They worked. Healthy bodies got us where we wanted to go. A chronic illness requires us to respect the limitations of our bodies, and at the same time, find ways to go on with our lives. Especially at the beginning, it is tempting to ignore symptoms and do things in spite of our bodies urging us not to. In the long run, these physical signals are best respected. Paying attention to the special needs of our bodies and simultaneously trying to live a normal life becomes a real challenge.

In addition to walking a tightrope between life's demands and bodily limitations, we have to live with lots of uncertainty and ambiguity. The meaning of lab tests is often unclear. "This could be something; maybe, maybe not," is a phrase people with chronic illness hear all too frequently. "Very often, mild and smoldering disease tends to remain so," says Dr. Stanley Pillemer of the Sjögren's Syndrome Clinic at the National Institutes of Health. "Even when tests are clearly positive, they may be of uncertain significance. It is important for patients to know that the treatments are quite similar across a variety of diagnoses. Although a specific diagnosis may be helpful and sometimes reassuring, it will do little to change the treatment. The physician will focus on the symptoms and signs of the disease and tailor the treatment according to the severity of the manifestations and the risks and benefit of the treatment" (Pillemer 2002).

It can be difficult to live with the unpredictability of what it all means and what aspects of life the disease will impact. "What will happen next?" and "Where will I be in five years?" are questions that are often asked by people with chronic illness. The underlying concern is impossible to miss.

Being a patient also means being thrown into a system of care that is often short on caring and stunning in its indifference. This gives us greater reason to search out the best people we can for our care. Increasingly, managed care provides limited choices and has introduced hard economics into the relationship between patient and physician. As medical consumers, we have the right to demand the best and take the time and energy to search out those physicians and other health care providers who will become both partners and allies. Human beings invariably disappoint each other sometimes, and in the doctor-patient relationship, like any other, there is a necessary give-and-take. Still, our doctors are our best allies in the medical world, and it is our responsibility to do what Max did: seek out the best people available to us and empower ourselves.

Sometimes it's easy to get fed up. In April 1997 Teri wrote the following in her journal:

> Yesterday, I had a mammogram, today is a rest day, and tomorrow I'll have an MRI. Last week, I saw my rheumatologist and now I'm waiting to see if I need an endoscopy. If I do, I'll have to see my gastroenterologist, whom I haven't seen since the Naprosyn I took burned a hole in my stomach, as if the lining of my stomach was a couch and a cigarette had been left burning. Next week I have an appointment with the orthopedist to interpret the MRI. So far this year, I've seen the ophthalmologist, dentist, dermatologist, gynecologist, internist, endocrinologist, and my rheumatologist. I'm fully expecting the orthopedist will refer me to a podiatrist, who will no doubt look at my feet and tell me that I need surgery if I expect to continue walking. It's only April, I'm just getting started. There are follow-up visits, more tests and procedures that my doctors tell me I should consider. I'm desperately trying to get the dog to the vet.

Frustration and impatience are par for the course. It's only human to give in. Sometimes, allowing ourselves to give in to these emotions is the only way to get through them and go on.

Humor, too, is a useful way to deal with the difficulties of having an illness. Ronald Berman, a California physician, recently described his own experience of being a patient:

> I managed to get through the procedure with aplomb, though they took everything else from me. When they had me stripped and in one of those backless gowns with all my possessions in a locker, the nurse looked at me and said, "We'll need your glasses and your wristwatch as well."
>
> "Do you have a drawer for my dignity?" I asked.
>
> She looked at the checklist on her clipboard and said, "We got that already."
>
> She was right, too (Berman 2001).

As this story illustrates, no one is spared. When it is possible, humor is a tool we can all use. Whether they like to admit it or not, sooner or later most physicians will become patients. When they do, they usually come away with a new respect and empathy for the experience.

Heal, Not Cure

Physicians who deal with chronic diseases are in the business of trying to heal when there is no cure. For much of history, physicians were in this position. Patients either got better, possibly through some intervention of the physician, or they died. Today, because of technological advances in the treatment of disease, people live longer and more productive lives, and they need to heal even when they cannot be cured.

We want to emphasize the healing nature of the doctor-patient relationship. The good doctor, as we have heard again and again, is a person who can put himself in someone else's shoes, listens carefully, and makes you feel that it is possible to speak about whatever is on your mind. A good doctor is an oasis in the experience of illness, a person with whom you can talk unreservedly and without hesitation or shame, a person who lightens the experience of living with a chronic disease.

Remember to always take an active role in your treatment. Be sure to do the following:

* Find the best physicians you can, the ones who feel "right" for you. Keep looking, even if this takes a while.

* Remember that there must be a good fit between the parties involved if there is to be a good working relationship.

* Talk to your physician about how to get in touch with him or her before there is an emergency, so you will know what to do. Have a plan. You may never need it, but it is a good feeling to know that it's there if you do.

* Make sure your physician knows all relevant information. When there are multiple medical problems, clear communication may take some organization on your part.

* Get medical records and copies of past lab tests if you need them. Ask for current lab results if you want them, so that you can keep your own medical records for reference.

* Educate yourself about Sjögren's syndrome and any other conditions you may have. Show your physician what you've been reading. Ask questions that are relevant to your own physical situation.

Remember that Sjögren's is a disease that varies greatly among individuals. Treatment will not be the same for everyone, although there are some standard treatments. Treatment will vary depending on the nature of the disease, your age, your overall physical health, and what other conditions are present. What your physician knows will allow him or her to create the best treatment plan possible, but no physician is infallible. If it isn't working, don't hesitate to say so.

Good doctors exist. We hope this chapter has offered proof of that. There are physicians who will go the extra mile and who strive to preserve the humanity of the healing tradition. They see their patients as whole people. They may not be the first physicians you encounter, but they are out there. The goal is to find them.

6

Reactions to Illness

Having a chronic illness presents a challenge that will last for the rest of your life. When Sjögren's is mild, you do not have to make many compromises or changes in lifestyle. The more severe the disease, the more adjustments you must make.

You might think that the more pervasive the illness, the more emotionally devastated a person would be, but this is not necessarily true. Some people have a very strong emotional reaction to mild or relatively mild illness. They are devastated and unable to function, while others who are very sick manage to retain their equanimity. The correlation between the degree of illness and the emotional reaction is not always a logical or rational one.

Many books on illness stress the importance of staying optimistic and positive, and we agree that a positive attitude and an optimistic outlook are both important and helpful. We also think that coping with illness presents a complex set of circumstances that can vary from day to day, hour to hour. Sometimes Sjögren's is merely annoying background noise, sometimes it is the cause of great distress, and sometimes it is overwhelming. Because this is true, we want to acknowledge that there are times when staying positive is difficult or impossible, and the best attitude in the world will not change this fact. Staying positive does not exclude getting anxious, angry, depressed, or scared. Having a fundamentally positive attitude may lead to a quicker recovery from periods of anxiety or depression, but it does not prevent anyone from experiencing these feelings in reaction to circumstances that are stressful, frightening, and anxiety provoking. You may have difficult times to get through, as if you are caught in an undertow and wondering when you will make it back to the safety of the shore.

In living with a chronic disease, it can be the little things that make all the difference in whether you are able to cope successfully or not (Kleinman 1988). A kind word, a hug, an awareness that someone cares, all impact the way you are able to cope with stressful situations.

Reactions to illness are made up of fluctuating emotional components. Sometimes one feeling predominates; at other times feelings are all mixed together, and it is difficult to sort them out.

How Coping Styles Differ

People cope with illness in very different ways. One person wants everyone to know what is happening to him, while another tells no one. One person is determined to live her life just as she did before she was aware of having any health problems at all, while another sees her illness as reason to give up and withdraw from the world. One person wants to know everything about his diagnosis, while another finds that even minimal information is too much to handle. One person is overwhelmed with emotion, while another shows no emotion at all. Some people are determined to take charge, while others see life spiraling out of control with no way to get it back.

How you cope with illness is probably consistent with how you generally cope with problems. It has a lot to do with your personality.

While we don't have room to go into personality theory here, what we can say is that the person who actively tries to explain and master the world is likely to do so when confronted by illness. The person who is passive and usually allows other people to make decisions for him or her is likely to continue this practice. If you have issues with trust, you are very likely to have a difficult time trusting your physicians. If you suffer from anxiety and depression, you may be more likely to experience these emotions than someone else who has no history of these conditions.

Illness can also be interpreted differently depending on the circumstances of your life and how you perceive major challenges. One person may see the illness as a sign from God, telling them that they must live their life in a more meaningful way; another sees it as a signal that all our lives are finite and it is time to set priorities and stick to them. One person becomes religious in response to the diagnosis, while another curses God and asks how this could have happened.

Sometimes the interpretation remains unconscious for months or years, as it did for Greta, who felt that she was deeply flawed because of her illness, and no one would want to be with her. She was sure her husband would leave her, although he never mentioned this as a possibility. She was convinced that he only stayed with her because he was an honorable man. During this period several of her friendships almost ended in disaster. Greta was unknowingly sending out signals that no one would want to be with her, unintentionally broadcasting her belief that this was so. Once she became aware of her feelings, she was able to change the way she saw herself and change the nature of her interactions. The meaning of her illness—that she was now deeply flawed—might have become a self-fulfilling prophecy. Fortunately, it did not.

If you experienced illness as a child or had an ill parent or sibling, you will likely have a different reaction from someone who has little or no previous experience with illness. Someone who was frightened by illness as a child may go to great lengths to deny his or her illness as an adult. Another person who watched helplessly as a parent or sibling lay ill may feel helpless in turn, or may respond by becoming an activist. Your life history and your interpretation of illness are bound together. They are the raw ingredients of a stew, although the resulting emotional and behavioral outcomes vary from person to person.

Other factors affect how you cope. An important one is the quality of your interpersonal relationships. If you feel that you can count on others, and that others will be there for you and support you, you are likely to have a very different experience of illness from a person who feels alone and without support. Age and stage of life make a difference too. Someone diagnosed with Sjögren's syndrome in her late fifties or sixties as she approaches retirement—who has achieved financial stability and has a husband, children, and even grandchildren who are able to help out—has reason to react differently from a woman in her twenties who is just beginning a career, or a woman in her early thirties about to have her first child, or a single woman with no one she can call on for support. We say *she*, but gender probably does not make much difference here; the same is true for men.

Illness cannot be separated from the context of your life. The way in which you react is a composite of your experiences, the severity of your illness, and the compromises it necessitates.

How to Be Resilient

We consider resilience a goal. Some people are naturally resilient; others must work to achieve it. Sometimes, when the disease is overwhelming, it is difficult to feel larger than the illness.

A chronic illness generates uncertainty, anxiety, frustration, and sometimes, depression. Periodically, you may ask "Why?" or, as one patient asked silently and out loud for at least the first ten years, "What do I do now, God, what am I supposed to do now?" Over time, for this patient, the nature of the question changed and it became less relevant. Life went on anyway, despite Sjögren's syndrome. She learned to modify her life, to do things in small increments, and to compromise, set goals, plan, and allow extra time for things.

Our culture places a great deal of emphasis on "not giving in" to illness. We agree that no one should give in too easily, but we think that what constitutes *too easily* is a personal decision. Sometimes, you have to give in. Illness necessitates change. Resilience means adapting. It does not mean carrying on with all normal activities and making your condition worse in the process. Resilience means being able to develop new strategies and new ways to cope with both familiar and unfamiliar situations. In a sense, a chronic illness makes it necessary to learn new ways to be.

Reactions to Diagnosis

If you have been symptomatic for years, going from physician to physician without learning what is wrong, a diagnosis can be a relief, or it can be very threatening. You may very well have mixed feelings. You may feel relieved and validated that there is really something wrong, that this is not all in your head, and feel a simultaneous sense of distress and concern. For many people, diagnosis confirms what they have known intuitively. The initial sense of validation then gives way to acknowledging that both your present and your future have changed. It may be difficult at first to think about the future or to make plans because you feel so much uncertainty.

A sense of shock and a period of grieving may accompany a diagnosis. Grieving for lost health may be a natural consequence of learning you have a chronic illness. You can be still be shocked, even if you already knew that there was really something wrong.

The Concept of Chronicity

If this is the first chronic health problem you have, the concept of a chronic disease may take a while (or a long time) to assimilate. Much of our experience with illness is that it is transient. With the flu, for example, you get better if you wait long enough. Sometimes health problems improve on their own. Sometimes they require medical or even surgical intervention, but ultimately, many health problems go away.

The fatigue and malaise of autoimmune diseases can feel very much like the flu. You have good days and bad days. Good days nurture the hope that the disease will not dominate your life. Even now, after so many years, many of us admit to wishfully thinking, "When I wake up, this disease will have gone away." Eventually you realize the disease is here to stay.

How Others React to You

As you know, it can be difficult to explain Sjögren's syndrome because most people have never heard of it. In answer to the question, "What's that?" you may explain that Sjögren's is a disease of dry eyes and dry mouth, or that it is a first cousin to lupus, or that it affects the moisture-producing glands, or that it is dryness, fatigue, arthritis, and muscle aches all rolled into one. In response, others often appear blank or vague. Many do not understand what kind of crisis having this little-known disease represents.

Most people do not understand what it means to have dry eyes and a dry mouth and think that it is not a very big deal. They may say, "Is that all?" and wonder what you are complaining about. They do not understand the pain of waking up with a scratched cornea or what it is like to be exquisitely sensitive to light. They have not experienced dry mouth or swollen parotid glands. They are unfamiliar with the fatigue that people experience with Sjögren's syndrome and the myriad of other symptoms that occur when other organs are affected. As a result, you may receive little sympathy.

Many people with Sjögren's do not appear to be sick. This increases the difficulty of getting others to take it seriously. "You can't look so well and feel so sick," is a refrain familiar to many patients with Sjögren's, lupus, and other autoimmune diseases. In fact, you may find that you tend to sleep more in the midst of a flare, with the result that you feel very sick but look rested and well.

Sjögren's syndrome is a disease of stability (sometimes remission) and exacerbation. Since there is no known cure, the goal is to create as much stability as possible, and to prevent the disease from getting worse. Crises can and do occur, however, in the form of organ involvement, infection, and exacerbation of the underlying autoimmune disease. In a medical sense, such crises need to be dealt with as swiftly as possible. In a psychological sense, you experience an increased sense of vulnerability. You are well one day, knowing that tomorrow may be a completely different experience. It may even feel as if the sword of Damocles is just above your head, hanging by a very slender thread about to break at any time. You wonder what will happen next.

Illness As Punishment

Illness can seem like a punishment when you've committed no crime. Some people wonder how God could let such a thing happen. They wonder whether they did something that brought on the illness. Then they want to know what they did.

Others blame their genes or the environment or the stress in their lives, and ask whether any or all of those things were instrumental in the development of their disease. Still others may accept that this is a part of life and that although there is no reason they should have developed a chronic illness, there is no real reason why they should not have, either.

Underlying many of these questions is the idea of a just world. The idea of a just world is, quite simply, that if you live a good and righteous life, a life where obligations and responsibilities are fulfilled, the world will be good to you in return. Suddenly, in the face of an illness or other crisis for which there is no explanation, the world is no longer just. Perhaps it never was, and the idea of a just world is something that people use to keep themselves feeling safe.

Look around. History and the newspapers are full of tragedy. Until something happens that touches us personally, however, these events are always things that happen to someone else. We protect ourselves by thinking that as long as we play by the rules, we will be all right. When something happens to us, we cross the line and join the ranks of those others who have also had bad things happen.

In his book, *When Bad Things Happen to Good People* (1981), Rabbi Harold S. Kushner says that there is only one question that really matters: "Why do bad things happen to good people?" There may be no answer, he says, but since we are human, we try to construct meaning and we search for answers. This is a book written by a man of faith who has known personal tragedy. Shortly after his third birthday, his son Aaron was diagnosed with a rare disease called progeria, which caused rapid aging. Aaron died in his early teens, and the book was the result of Kushner's questions and grief over his son's life and premature death. This is a book for everyone, regardless of religious persuasion, or whether you believe in God. Bad things do happen. When they happen, being human, we want to know why.

Who's to Blame?

"Did I do this to myself?" is a question you may ask. Perhaps the question is associated with feelings of guilt, as if something you did might have directly or indirectly caused you to get sick. Anecdotally, it does seem that many people with Sjögren's experienced the onset of disease following a period of intense or prolonged stress—a divorce, the death of a parent, the loss of a job—although this is not always the case. Was there something in your reaction to these stressful life events that caused your body to produce a disease? Or was the predisposition to disease there, waiting for a period when you were particularly vulnerable, to manifest itself? We do not believe you are responsible for your disease. Why does one person have a heart attack, another a stroke, or why does one person develop cancer and someone else an autoimmune disease? Perhaps in the future we will know more about the etiology of autoimmune diseases and will be able to answer these questions with increased certainty.

Though we don't have the answer to these questions, we do know that there are things you can do to manage your life and live in the best way possible. There are things you can take control of, and you should make every effort to do so. It is important to remember that autoimmune diseases send out subtle signals for years, and that many of these go unnoticed. You cannot know exactly or even approximately when your illness began. Sjögren's may manifest itself after a prolonged divorce or the loss of a parent, but the disease process may actually have started years before the period of stress began. A period of prolonged stress may accelerate and exacerbate the disease, which creates an appearance of cause and effect between the two.

Expectations and Disappointment

People whose lives have been compromised by illness can feel that they are not living up to their own expectations. Having Sjögren's syndrome may mean giving up the old image you had of yourself, of things you thought you would do and ways you would live your life. It is easy to feel deprived and cheated. Some people feel guilty that they are not using their skills or training. Some feel dissatisfied and discouraged. You may need to face the loss of previous expectations before you can achieve new ways of seeing yourself in the world.

What to Do Now

No one grew up with plans to have a chronic disease. It just happens. Once it does, you have to do everything possible to live in the best way you can.

"What do I do now?" is a question that can be asked in different ways. It can be asked in desperation, grief, or sorrow. It can be asked as a way of acknowledging the reality that something has happened and it is necessary to go forward. The answers often appear over time, as you learn what it means for you to live with Sjögren's syndrome.

It is easier to answer the question if you ask it slightly differently: "What must I do in order to deal with the problems I am having?" "What treatments are there?" "How do I find them?" "Which doctor should I see first?" All of these questions imply a take-charge approach. When you don't feel well, it can sometimes be difficult to get mobilized, but in all probability, it has never been more important. If things seem overwhelming, break down whatever needs to be done into small components. Take baby steps, but keep on going.

Figuring out what to do takes time. If you don't feel well one day, do what you can, and put off what you can't do. But be persistent.

Here are some answers to the question, "What do I do now?":

* Find a physician you can work with, one who understands the nature of Sjögren's syndrome.

* Educate yourself about Sjögren's.

* Find out what resources there are in your community.

* Join the Sjögren's Syndrome Foundation.

* Try different medications until you find ones that work for you. Sometimes the side effects are as bad as the symptoms, but when medication works, you *will* feel better.

* Begin to think about what changes having Sjögren's necessitates, including changes in the way you manage your home, family, work, friends, and other relationships.

* Seek less stress and more rest. A good diet and moderate exercise do help to make you feel better. Depending on what your life is like when you are diagnosed, it may feel as if reducing stress is impossible. Look for ways to make small changes.

* Seek whatever support you need. Don't be shy or hesitant about this. Nothing is too small or inconsequential to ask about, if it bothers you.

* Focus on the things you can do. Keep trying things until you find something that makes you feel satisfied with yourself. One small thing will lead to others. It is very important to stay positive and not give up. If you feel discouraged, take a break and start again.

Sometimes it is hard to be satisfied with life while adapting to the changes in your body. Healthy people can take their bodies for granted. They know their limits and how far they can push themselves. You may not know what you can do from day to day or even within a day.

It may be necessary to make compromises. Part of the answer to "What do I do now?" has to do with paying close attention to the way the disease reacts when you do certain things. If, by experience, you learn that doing everything on your "to do list" makes you feel worse, make the necessary adjustments:

* Prioritize, and if need be, prioritize again, depending on how you feel. Do the things that are most important first. Give yourself an extension if necessary.

* Set goals for what you want to accomplish.

* Take small steps and be persistent.

* If you are someone who has always done things at the last minute, think seriously about not procrastinating. Give yourself time so that if you need to take a break, you can.

Different people with Sjögren's have different limits. Don't judge yourself against anyone except yourself. Do as much as you can without doing too much. Yes, there is a very fine line to be walked.

Illness, Not Metaphor

In *Illness As Metaphor,* Susan Sontag points out that "Illness is the night-side of life, a more onerous citizenship. Everyone who is born holds dual citizenship, in the kingdom of the well and in the kingdom of the sick. Although we all prefer to use only the good passport, sooner or later each of us is obliged, at least for a spell, to identify ourselves as citizens of that other place" (1977, 3).

Illness, according to Sontag, is common to all. The simplest way to be ill is to be ill without adding meaning, because doing so causes additional distress. At the time the book was written, Sontag was swimming against the tide. A number of studies tried to show that certain characteristics, especially feelings of hopelessness and helplessness and despair, were associated with the development of different kinds of diseases, especially cancer. Many of these studies used small numbers of people who were already ill when the studies began, making it difficult to distinguish which feelings had actually preceded the illness and which had followed.

In *Illness As Metaphor,* Sontag talks about how tuberculosis was once thought of as a disease caused by an excess of romantic passion. In the nineteenth century, it was thought that people became ill because life was intolerable to them, and on some level, perhaps unknowingly, they wished to die in order to avoid such intolerable pain. As Sontag eloquently points out, this kind of thinking was forced to change once it was discovered that the real cause of tuberculosis was a bacillus and that the disease could be treated with antibiotics. We have seen cancer (and perhaps autoimmune diseases) also described as failures of living. Nothing could be more punitive, she says. The simplest way to be ill is to be ill without giving the illness additional meaning. Otherwise, you are twice punished, once by the illness and once by feeling in some way responsible for your condition.

We are impressed by the inherent wisdom in this. Especially at times when Sjögren's is worse, or during any illness-related crisis, we have found that the best way to cope is to deal with the problems, and put energy into getting better.

7

Riding a Roller
Coaster of Emotions

We have said that no two people react to having Sjögren's syndrome in quite the same way. Some are so busy coping with the physical aspects of the disease that they are only minimally impacted by its emotional consequences. Others ride an emotional roller coaster and experience depression, anxiety, and other overwhelming emotions. Physicians often fail to ask about the emotional impact of Sjögren's, or ask in only the most superficial way. Sometimes it seems as if no one really wants to know.

In this chapter, we describe the range of different emotions and their relationship to having Sjögren's syndrome. You will find sections on withdrawal, deprivation and envy, guilt, shame, and frustration. There are also descriptions of the denial, boredom, anger, grief, anxiety, depression, and stress that are engendered by living with chronic illness. They are not in any particular order. You may have experienced many or all of these emotions, or only a few of them.

There is an important relationship between emotion and coping. An emotional reaction to an event combines feelings with cognitive components. The way you interpret an event (cognitively) will impact the way you feel. For example, your perception of an event as threatening may make you anxious, angry, or alarmed. Someone who experiences the same event as benign is less likely to feel the same way. In turn, the way you think is influenced by the way you feel. If you are anxious about a situation, you will see it in a different way than if you are calm. This helps explain why each person's reaction is so individualized, yet it would be a mistake to assume that there is no commonality of experience. There is often an immediate sense of relief and recognition when two perfect strangers with Sjögren's meet and begin to talk.

Withdrawal

It is easy to isolate yourself when you do not feel well or when you feel tired and are in pain. It can feel as if it takes too much energy to do anything. You may want to go somewhere, but it takes all your energy just to get ready to go and you arrive at your destination exhausted, while everyone else arrives with energy and enthusiasm. It makes you feel different. When you feel this way, it can feel as if it is just easier to be by yourself.

Withdrawal is sometimes a good response when it gives you a chance to recharge, but in the extreme, it can make things worse to isolate yourself from friends and family. Withdrawal may be a form of self-protection. If you withdraw, you cannot be criticized for your inability to do something. It can also be a way of protecting others. If you withdraw, you don't have to worry about burdening others. You simply keep to yourself. A sense of isolation may be the result of anxiety and depression. In turn, anxiety and depression cause even more isolation.

The fact is, you need people, especially when you are sick. When you feel your worst, you need the people you care for most, the people with whom you are most at ease. These are the people who keep you grounded.

Even when you are very sick, you have something to give to others, something they would miss if you were to isolate yourself and withdraw. You can listen, console, and give advice. You can lend an ear when your child tells you about his or her day at school, or sympathize with a partner who has had a bad day at work. You can give someone a hug. You may not have enough energy to hike, work out, or make dinner, but by staying connected, you can sustain your emotional ties.

Deirdre is a good example of someone who has been able to avoid isolation and withdrawal. Once an active counselor who accompanied her husband on frequent business trips, she can no longer fly and now gets around with the help of a scooter because of lupus and Sjögren's syndrome. She is sometimes unable to shop or make dinner for her family. When asked how she feels about this, she said that while she is naturally frustrated by what she is unable to do, she feels that she is still a help to her husband. She is involved with her children and grandchildren, and when she can, she works to educate her community about autoimmune disease. Through the Internet, she keeps in touch with people all over the world. Life is not what she planned, but she has stayed connected.

Deprivation and Envy

Envy is a feeling that contains anger. Usually, it is anger about something that is desired but cannot be obtained. It is connected to deprivation when someone else has something you want that is unavailable to you, such as health. It is easy to envy people with healthy bodies and to feel deprived when your illness makes it impossible for you to do the things you were able to do and still want to do.

Some people feel that a sense of deprivation is formed early in life (Gaylin 1984) and that it may be reactivated by later events, including illness. Deprivation is worse when we feel that something, or the possibility of something, has been taken away and will not return (Gaylin 1984).

Guilt

There are different kinds of guilt applicable to living with a chronic illness, as we mentioned in chapter 6. The first has to do with feeling that you have done something bad, and the illness is retribution for some past sin or crime. This kind of guilt is connected to the question, "What did I ever do to deserve this?" The implication is, "This illness is my punishment."

The second form of guilt is related to not feeling good enough, as in not living up to your own expectations for yourself. This kind of guilt may occur after you have lived with your illness for a while and notice changes in lifestyle occurring because of it.

The third form of guilt is a variant of the first. It is the feeling that you must have done something to bring this illness on yourself. There is a large amount of literature that suggests there is a disease-prone personality (Hafen et al. 1996). We want to emphasize that we dislike this way of thinking. It suggests that illness is the result of an ineffectual way of being in the world or results from having certain personality traits.

Guilt is an emotion that can be difficult to recognize and tolerate. Because of this, it is sometimes transformed into anger and projected outward as blame.

Shame

Shame, like guilt, is a very private emotion. It is invisible and often not recognized unless it is overwhelming. People with any kind of an illness are at risk for both shame and humiliation because they may experience their disease as a defect (Lazare 1987). Anyone who has ever been a patient has experienced the exposure that comes with immersion in the medical system. People are literally stripped of their clothes, and as Dr. Ronald Berman (2001) pointed out in chapter 5, they are often stripped of their dignity as well. Like guilt, shame and humiliation may both be felt as anger. Angry patients are more likely to withhold information from their physicians and to complain and file lawsuits (Lazare 1987).

Frustration

The lack of consistency in the lives of people with Sjögren's syndrome cannot be underestimated. The fluctuations created by this disease are enough to drive the most stable person crazy. One minute you feel quite well, ready to tackle anything; an hour later, you are exhausted, unable to move. Bad days make it difficult to plan, and not being able to count on your body to behave with regularity makes life difficult.

The kind of frustration that comes from chronic illness has to do with the everyday things that are changed and limited by the illness. The sense of limitation that many people feel for the first time is difficult to deal with. When you have limited energy, it is hard to get everything done. Some people are unable to do the physical things they once enjoyed: hiking, running, or even gardening. Work, friends, hobbies, hopes, and dreams may need to be curtailed. It can be incredibly frustrating to have to give something up when you want to keep doing it, when it is something you have enjoyed doing, or something that is necessary (like work) to sustain your quality of life.

Interpersonal relationships can also be sources of frustration as well as comfort. Colleagues, friends, or even relatives who just cannot seem to understand what Sjögren's is all about can frustrate you. For years, whenever Lily would tell family members that she wasn't feeling very well, their answer was always the same. "What's wrong?" her relatives would say, in chorus. Lily would answer, with as much patience as she could muster, "I have a disease which makes me feel unwell much of the time. It's called Sjögren's syndrome." They never understood. Eventually she prepared herself for their inadequate response and felt less frustrated.

Frustration with Health Care

Many people find their immersion in the medical system frustrating. Everything from appointment secretaries who are rude to long waits for doctor's appointments can be difficult when you are not feeling well. Medical practices seem to create the feeling of "hurry up and wait." Patients are told to check in a half hour before their appointment, only to find that "the doctor is running late." It is indeed frustrating to have to wait several months for an appointment, then find that the doctor's attention is elsewhere, or that the appointment yields no helpful or new information. In many managed care systems, each referral to a specialist requires authorization from a primary care physician, so that access is limited. In such circumstances, an appointment that is unsatisfactory is particularly frustrating, since it is not just a matter of picking up the phone and rescheduling with someone else. Sometimes, when many different specialists are involved in your care, you feel like a Ping-Pong ball bounced back and forth between different doctors, with no one ultimately responsible, and it is easy to fall through the cracks.

Dealing with Frustration

As we said earlier, each person has his or her own unique way of coping with difficult life events. One person deals with frustration by going for a walk, one by meditating, one uses humor. Someone else gets angry, and another person turns to alcohol.

No one is perfect. We all have our good and bad days. We can cope with something one day that becomes impossible two days later, or even an hour later (Kleinman 1988). This is completely normal. Each of us can tolerate a certain level of frustration, and that level varies from day to day, hour to hour.

You probably cope better when you are not tired, when you feel that there are people who can support you, and when you do not feel overwhelmed with what you need to do. Sometimes small things may enable you to cope or not; a fight with a spouse or a word of praise from a supervisor may sway the situation in opposite directions. When a husband leaves with an "I love you" in the morning, it can generate strength to face the day. When a couple parts with harsh words, they cause stress that makes it difficult to cope with both illness and other matters that day.

Some suggestions for coping with frustration are:

* Do difficult things at whatever time of day you feel best.

* Take a break and do something that gives you pleasure.

* Go out with a friend.

* Do something completely different.

* If you feel overwhelmed by something, do what you can, then go on to something else. You can always return to it later.

* Exercise.

There are lots of things to do in this world. No one has to do everything. Even with Sjögren's syndrome, there are many things you can do. Figure out what you can do each day. Try to do that much and no more.

Denial

Denial is a way of hiding something, even from yourself. It is one way of responding to a threatening situation over which you perceive yourself to have little or no control. Denial can be a protective mechanism that enables you to absorb information or accept a new reality slowly, on your own terms. It can be harmful when it prevents you from seeking help or getting treatment.

With regard to a difficult diagnosis, an acute illness, or surgery, some denial may prevent you from being overwhelmed or incapacitated. After surgery, it may be more important to recover than to understand all the implications of a diagnosis immediately. Even when difficult decisions need to be made, there is usually a little time to assimilate information. Some people have a great need to know, while others actually do better with just a little information. They do not need to read everything that has been written on Sjögren's; for them, less is more.

Denial in illness-related matters might be subtle. A person may appreciate the fact that she has an illness but fail to react or make any changes because of it. One of us responded to her diagnosis by thinking, "I'll just have to try harder to get everything done." She made minor concessions and scraped by for a few years, until she had to make significant modifications to her lifestyle so that her illness was in better control.

The opposite of denial is to place the illness at the center of your life and make it the way you define yourself. Every interpersonal encounter then becomes an opportunity to discuss the disease. Although it may certainly feel like it is at the center of your life, remember that you are more than your Sjögren's or any other illness.

Boredom

Few healthy people realize how boring illness can be. Boredom is the absence of activity, passion, and interest. When you are bored, time elongates and passes slowly. Gaylin (1979) says that we experience boredom not as a threat to survival, but to the value of survival. Boredom is a feeling associated with lassitude and physical malaise. The desire to get up and do something may be there; you may know what you would like to do, but you lack the energy to do it.

You may suffer from boredom during an enforced period of rest while you wait for a flare to pass and for energy to return. Perhaps there is an initial sense of relief at not having to do anything, but when a period of inactivity is prolonged, you would probably prefer to be doing something that interests you.

Anger

Anger is not one emotion, but a range of emotions. We say we are angry when we are irritated, annoyed, resentful, furious, or impatient (Gaylin 1979). Anger may be a response to envy, betrayal, threat, deprivation, guilt, or injustice (Gaylin 1984), and it may be a response to all these feelings associated with Sjögren's syndrome. If you feel angry, it is difficult to know how to express it. Should you be angry with yourself, your genes, your body, the stress in your life, your husband or partner? The list of possibilities is endless. Because there is no easy answer to this question, you may direct your anger inward, or at those around you.

It can be difficult to express anger at authority figures or at people you need. Expressing anger is especially hard for women, who, according to Harriet Lerner (1997) have not been allowed to have angry feelings. A physician who doesn't call back may make his patient angry, but the patient may be hesitant to get angry at the physician because she needs him. Lerner says that women often wait until their anger passes or until it escalates to a level where they can no longer control it. When anger cannot be expressed directly, people may become passive-aggressive or blaming, or express their feelings in other inappropriate ways. The angry patient may "forget" to show up for a scheduled appointment. Someone feeling angry about having a disease that restricts what she can do may not discuss her limitations, but she may get angry at something else instead.

Angry feelings in the present may bring up angry feelings from the past. A patient whose physician has not responded may feel "he doesn't like me" and have the same experience he or she had as a child with a parent who withdrew affection. The patient may decide never to see this physician again and express his or her anger by going to someone else. An alternate response, and one that might be more satisfying, would be to discuss the situation and see if it could be resolved. On the other hand, repeated feelings of anger after seeing a physician may be an important clue that something is not right in the relationship.

Anger and Medication

Some medications, such as prednisone, may cause personality changes, which include irritability and depression.

Normal versus Pathological Anger

How do you know if you are too angry? It can be difficult to differentiate normal from pathological anger. Here are some general guidelines:

* Normal anger usually has a cause and is in proportion to that cause (Mazer 2001).

* Anger as a response to every situation is problematic and may be pathological.

* Anger that is abusive and ends in aggression or violence is pathological.

* Anger that is the source of self-destructive behavior is pathological.

* Repeated angry confrontations that fail to change anything are problematic.

* Anger displaced on to "safe" figures, such as a spouse or a child, is problematic and may seriously damage those relationships.

Illness-Related Angry Feelings

What is the best way to cope with angry feelings?

* Distance yourself. Take time and think about what makes you angry. Consider constructive ways to deal with the situation so that you do not repeat the same thing again and again.

* Find ways to distract yourself and diffuse your anger.

* Find other people who can share your feelings in a constructive setting such as a support group. If no such group is available in your area, there are Internet groups specifically for Sjögren's syndrome (see Resources).

* Monitor angry thoughts and feelings. Remember that feeling angry or thinking angry thoughts does not mean you have

to act on them. Take the time to figure out productive ways to translate thoughts and feelings into action.

Grief and Loss

Early in the course of your disease, any real losses may be in the future, but the sense of loss and grief can be very much in the present. The feelings of loss and grief may be mild or they may be disorganizing. They can be as powerful as when a loved one dies.

Grief may cause depression, but grief and depression are not synonymous. Grieving may occur as a perfectly normal reaction to the diagnosis of a chronic illness. Usually, people grieve over time, not at any one time. They do not grieve and "get over it." They grieve, go on with their lives, and then, when something else happens, they grieve again.

Grief is personal, easy to hide, and difficult to share. In the context of Sjögren's syndrome, it is sometimes difficult for friends and family to understand what you are going through. They see you up and about, doing things, carrying on with life, and they don't understand what has changed. They try, but don't get it. When this happens, you may feel invisible and unseen. It makes it all the more important to find people with whom you can share your feelings.

Some people find it easier to move on, or accept their illness and live with it, than others. Some never seem to experience grief or grieving. Some people may seem to adjust immediately to a new situation and find that their grief is deferred or postponed.

Anxiety

Common symptoms of anxiety are cold, clammy hands, feeling tremulous, dry mouth, sweating, nausea, muscle tension, and trouble swallowing (APA 2000). Of course, if you have dry mouth and trouble swallowing because you have Sjögren's syndrome, it may be easy to mistake one for the other! Anxiety is both an emotion and a clinical entity. It may be a perfectly normal reaction to a life-changing event, or anxiety may present in ways that are also life limiting, such as phobias, panic attacks, post-traumatic stress, and generalized anxiety. Sometimes anxiety is mixed with depression, and the line between the two is very thin. Some people experience anxiety in their bodies. Given the vague nature of Sjögren's syndrome, especially in the early stages, many people have been told that they are suffering from anxiety. The irony here is that they may be anxious because they know something is wrong with them but no one seems to know what it is.

What are people with Sjögren's syndrome anxious about? You may be anxious about the disease progressing, being incapacitated, being dependent on others, losing the ability to work and earn a living, experiencing financial problems, loss of self-esteem, changes in your sense of self, and changes in your relationships, to name a few reasons.

Uncertainty associated with lab test results is one anxiety-provoking aspect of living with Sjögren's syndrome. We have repeatedly been impressed by how much anxiety is the result of human interaction and human carelessness or error. Perhaps your doctor does not know exactly what certain test results mean. She or he may get a consultation, which takes time, but instead of telling you that, your call for results goes unanswered. You were supposed to get the results on Monday, and now it is Wednesday and you still don't know what is happening. You get anxious. In another scenario, the test is unclear, so your doctor wants to repeat it, but this raises your anxiety.

Don't wait until this kind of situation arises. Ask your doctor ahead of time to share the results of whatever lab tests you are having that might make you anxious. Set up an appointment if necessary. Ask your doctor to call you and explain the results even if they are not definitive. You are essentially asking your doctor to share the uncertainty with you. It may not give you the answer that you want, but it's better than dealing with the situation on your own.

People sometimes develop illness-related anxieties. They may become afraid to travel, because appropriate medical care may not be available. They may become afraid that doctors will not take them seriously or respond to them when they need help. Some people become anxious about what the illness will do to their marriage or relationship, and worry that they have passed the illness on to their children or grandchildren and that future generations will be affected. We are sure that this list is by no means exhaustive. Just the presence of an illness is enough to cause anxiety.

Does anyone live without anxiety? Maybe, but neither of us has ever met them. Some anxiety is a normal part of life. Problems arise when anxiety increases to the point where it interferes with normal living.

Vigilance, Worry, and Catastrophizing

Anxious people are vigilant. People who are vigilant fall into a range, from being on the lookout for new signs and symptoms, to those who are always taking their physical and emotional temperatures. Such vigilance may be part of an effort to control what is happening and is an attempt to catch any new developments in their earliest stage. In the extreme, vigilance is exhausting.

People who fall into the category of excessive worriers are likely to catastrophize. Catastrophizing is a process that convinces you that the worst is about to happen. You then react as if this were the actual case. When you catastrophize, an abnormal lab result is the first sign of a terminal illness. An increase in fatigue is sure to mean the onset of a flare or something worse. Someone who sneezes on the bus will definitely transmit a serious infection. Reassurance provides little or no relief from this kind of anxiety.

Sometimes this kind of thinking can be unlearned with experience. After many abnormal lab results, you begin to get a sense of what they mean. When you repeatedly feel sick, it may take too much energy to mount a full-scale alarm each time it happens. You come to understand what you feel and are able to take a more moderate, "I'll wait and see" approach. You can learn to monitor your thoughts and recognize when you are catastrophizing.

Generalized Anxiety

In order to be diagnosed with generalized anxiety, a person must experience apprehension for most of the time during a six-month period, and find it difficult to control the worry. In addition, the anxiety and worry are associated with at least three of the following symptoms:

1. Restlessness or feeling keyed up or on edge

2. Being easily fatigued

3. Difficulty concentrating or mind going blank

4. Irritability

5. Muscle tension

6. Sleep disturbance (difficulty falling or staying asleep, or rest-less unsatisfying sleep) (APA 2000, 476)

Many of these criteria overlap with those of Sjögren's and other autoimmune diseases. Seeing them may make it easier to under-stand why, in the absence of specific diagnostic signs, people with many different autoimmune diseases are so frequently told they are suffering from an anxiety disorder.

We understand only too well what it means to be told that "it is all in your head." If the problem is truly physiological, applying a psychological explanation will do nothing to alleviate the underlying causes.

Anxiety and Medical Conditions

A variety of endocrine or cardiovascular conditions cause anxi-ety and these may be associated with Sjögren's syndrome. Some medications also increase anxiety. A physician must first establish the medical condition, then determine if anxiety is the result of the dis-ease. Anxiety symptoms that are psychological in nature, and are in reaction to having Sjögren's syndrome, are considered to be an adjustment disorder with anxious (and depressed) mood. This is a common diagnosis among people with chronic illnesses.

Treating Illness-Related Anxiety

The treatment of anxiety depends on the nature of the anxiety, its intensity, and the identified reasons. The treating physician or therapist first has to determine the relationship of the anxiety to the illness. Does the person have a history of anxiety symptoms, or did the anxiety develop after the illness? If so, is it a psychological reac-tion to the illness or the result of organic causes? Once these ques-tions are answered, treatment plans can begin. There are mind-body programs for people with physical illnesses that teach the relaxation response (see chapter 10). Psychotherapy can be used to help an individual regain some sense of control.

Anxiety also may be treated with cognitive and behavioral programs designed to control stress and teach people to modify their responses to anxiety-provoking situations, or it may be treated with medications, or with some combination of these modalities.

Antianxiety medications (anxiolytics) in the benzodiazepine class: diazepam (Valium), clonazepam (Klonopin), and alprazolam (Xanax), are used in the treatment of panic attacks and generalized anxiety, as well as anxiety symptoms that do not meet the criteria for generalized anxiety (such as adjustment disorder). Valium is also useful as a muscle relaxant, while Klonopin has been found to be effective in the treatment of panic disorders (Medical Economics Company 2001). Xanax is used in the treatment of both generalized anxiety and panic disorder. Like all medications, benzodiazepines have side effects, may increase fatigue and dryness, and it may be necessary to try more than one before finding the correct medication for you. Medications in this class may cause dependence with long-term use. Just because one medication produces side effects or is ineffective does not mean that others in the same class will have similar results.

Antidepressants are increasingly used to treat both anxiety and depression. Like anxiolytics, antidepressants have a variety of side effects, including increased fatigue, agitation, constipation, nausea, and loss of libido. Some of these are transient and wear off as your body gets used to the medication. Both antianxiety and antidepressant medications increase dryness, but many people with Sjögren's are able to use them. Antidepressants have also been useful in the management of chronic pain.

Depression

You may respond to the uncertainty and limitations of Sjögren's syndrome with depression. Depression is not just sadness that doesn't go away. It is a much more complicated entity. People with depression can be irritable, fatigued, have little or no affect (emotion), have a diminished interest in sex, eat all the time, or have no appetite whatsoever. Depression makes it impossible to concentrate or make decisions. Some people sleep too much, others not at all. There is a feeling that life is not worth living or a feeling of worthlessness. In bipolar depression, people may have episodes of rapid thought processes, times when they are constantly in motion, have little or no need for sleep, and may become more reckless.

Depression may be a response to the loss of ability or loss of activity. It can be a reaction to changes in lifestyle and your sense of self. It can also be a response to chronic pain and sleep deprivation due to being in pain. Some people are more prone to depression than others, and as with autoimmune diseases, depression tends to run in families. It is possible that tendencies toward certain patterns of neurochemical responses are inherited and predispose some people to depression.

Theories of Depression

There are biological, psychological, and sociological theories of depression. Depression has been attributed both to the experience of loss and separation in childhood and the result of a neurochemical imbalance. Depression may be acute or chronic, overwhelming or mild. It may be tolerable or so intolerable that it leads to suicidal behavior (and suicide). It is definitely not something that can be willed away. Most people who get depressed would do anything to feel better if they could. Depression is not a moral failure. Depressed people are not "weak" in any sense of the word. Like anxiety, depression may be a consequence of an event, a symptom of a clinical syndrome, an emotion, or a complex disorder.

All of us are familiar with depression as an emotion. The differential diagnosis between a mood state and a clinical entity is sometimes difficult to make. It is safe to say that the majority of people have experienced feelings of depression at one time or another. Some people live with a low level of depressed mood throughout their lives.

To sum up, depression may be a chemical imbalance, a lifelong problem, a way of seeing the world, a conditioned pattern of response, a transient emotion, a sustained mood, a symptom of another disease, or a member of a group of disorders called mood disorders. It may be the result of being in chronic pain or living with an illness that robs you of your feeling of usefulness and eats away at your sense of self and self-esteem. It may be more than one of the above, as these categories are not mutually exclusive.

As researchers understand more about the connections between the brain and the immune system, with investigative techniques unavailable even twenty or thirty years ago, they are beginning to understand the connections between autoimmune diseases and depression. Instead of taking a blaming approach, such as, "You are a depressive person and your disease is the result of those feelings," they are beginning to understand that there may be a certain predisposition to both inflammatory disease and depression (Sternberg 2001).

Who Gets Depressed?

According to some researchers, nearly one-fourth of all women suffer clinical depression. Approximately 10 percent of the population in the United States suffers from major depression at any given time (7 percent women, 3 percent men). Another 4 to 5 percent of the population suffers depression that does not meet the criteria for a major depressive disorder but meets other clinical criteria (Hafen et al. 1996). Researchers also say that these figures are higher in winter, when a number of people suffer from seasonal affective disorder. People who have suffered an episode of major depression before being diagnosed with a chronic illness are more likely to suffer a recurrence.

Chronic illness may also cause or exacerbate lower levels of depression. People who become depressed as a reaction to their illness are considered to have an adjustment disorder with depressed mood. This kind of depression develops in direct response to a specific stress factor, such as the diagnosis of Sjögren's syndrome. Dysthymic disorder is a depression that is of a lower level than a major depression, but not necessarily in response to a specific life event. It may be chronic and people may live with it for years. We encourage people who feel they may be depressed to seek professional help. Depression is something that happens, and should be treated just like anything else when it does. As depression has come to be understood in terms of biological phenomena, some of the stigma previously attached to it has diminished.

Major Depression

The American Psychiatric Association (APA 2000) has established the following guidelines for diagnosing a major depressive episode:

Five (or more) of the following symptoms have been present during the same two-week period and represent a change from previous functioning; at least one of the symptoms is either (1) depressed mood or (2) loss of interest or pleasure.

Note: Do not include symptoms that are clearly due to a general medical condition.

1. depressed mood most of the day, nearly every day

2. markedly diminished interest or pleasure in all, or almost all activities, most of the day, nearly every day

3. significant weight loss or gain (e.g., a change of more than 5 percent of body weight in a month)

4. insomnia or hypersomnia nearly every day

5. psychomotor agitation or retardation nearly every day (observable by others, not merely subjective feelings of restlessness or being slowed down)

6. fatigue or loss of energy nearly every day

7. feelings of worthlessness or excessive or inappropriate guilt (which may be delusional) nearly every day

8. diminished ability to think or concentrate, or indecisiveness, nearly every day

9. recurrent thoughts of death or recurrent suicidal ideation (356)

Depression has been associated with sleep deprivation, fibromyalgia, and chronic pain, all familiar to people with autoimmune disease. Feelings of helplessness and hopelessness may occur in reaction to the limitations imposed by the illness, the uncertainty, and the general distress that accompanies Sjögren's syndrome. This is why therapy that helps regain a sense of control and helps overcome feelings of helplessness and hopelessness is so important.

Suicidality and Chronic Illness

Both depression and chronic illness can rob people of their sense of the future. Suicidal thoughts and feelings should always be taken seriously, even if they are transient, but especially when they are sustained with a well-formatted plan. Some questions to ask if you or someone you know may have suicidal feelings are:

- Do you have suicidal thoughts, i.e. have you thought that you do not want to live?

- Are these thoughts persistent and frequent? Are they present all or most of the time? Are you distressed by them? If not, do you find them compelling? Does suicide seem like a way out of present distress? Does it seem like the only way out?

- Have you lost hope for the future? Do you see a future for yourself?

- Are your suicidal thoughts specific; do you think about a specific way of committing suicide?

- Do you have the means to carry out your suicidal thoughts?

- Have you made any suicide attempts in the past?

A positive answer to any of these indicates that you or someone you know is at risk; the more positive answers, the more at risk a person is. If you feel that you or someone you know falls into this category, we urge you to get help immediately. Help may come from a primary care physician, therapist, mental health center, or, as a last resort, from the nearest emergency room of a local hospital.

One of the characteristics of major depression is that it engulfs and envelops a person completely, so there appears to be no way out of the pain. In addition to a sense of the future, perspective is lost in depression. It feels like depression is all there is, all there ever will be, and it will never go away. Fortunately, not all depression is this severe. People who have had a major depression and have recovered from it are often afraid of becoming depressed again and may become particularly distressed when they feel depression returning.

Depression and Disease

Are people with more serious disease more depressed? The answer is, not necessarily, according to research that Teri did a number of years ago. She interviewed women with breast cancer. The expectation was that the women with more widespread disease would be more depressed.

The results of this study showed that the severity of the disease was not a factor in how depressed the women were. What *was* significant was the quality of their support systems. The women who felt more supported, who felt that their friends and family accepted them without reservation, were less depressed than those who did not have this kind of support. While the study was done with cancer patients, the connection between depression and social support is an important one that should not be overlooked.

Getting Treatment

There are many different ways of treating depression and the proper treatment very much depends on the nature of the depression. The most important thing is to do something! Taking an active approach can be difficult when you are depressed, but it is absolutely necessary. When you are depressed, you don't feel like doing anything. The light at the end of the tunnel may be far away, but with some action, it becomes visible. It is important to get help. If you feel that you are unable to get help for yourself, tell someone how you feel and ask them to help you get started.

There are many different approaches to treating depression, from cognitive therapy to supportive and interpretive psychotherapy. Cognitive therapy focuses on the negative and self-deprecating thoughts that contribute to depression and utilizes the premise that if you can modify these underlying thoughts (and the behaviors that go along with them), changes in mood will follow. Cognitive therapy enables the individual to recognize negative thoughts that are present and influence behavior that may not be perceived or identified. Cognitive therapists also help identify feelings that go along with negative thoughts and usually focus on events in the present.

Some forms of psychotherapy for depression focus on the connection between past experience of loss and disappointment and the recapitulation of those feelings in the present. However, not all psychotherapy focuses on the past; much work can be done with a focus on the present. Supportive psychotherapy helps find ways to bolster your own coping strategies.

For someone whose depression is persistent and intense, a combination of medication and talk therapy is probably most effective. There are now numerous antidepressants that are chemically different, so it is usually possible to find one that works and has min-imal side effects. Most antidepressants require a trial period of sev-eral weeks, and you may need to try more than one drug; the wait for an effective and tolerable medication can be frustrating. It is hard to be patient when you are in pain, and this applies to emotional as well as physical pain. Learning what works for you and what you can do is a huge step in the right direction. The most important thing to remember is that depression can be treated.

Stress

According to Dr. Hans Selye (1974), one of the pioneers in stress research, stress is universal and unavoidable. When we talk about stress, we are actually referring to excessive stress, or a state of "distress."

We all have certain constitutional strengths and weaknesses. When combined with our early learning experiences, these may account for the way our bodies respond to stressful life events. Since our response to stress is filtered through our experience, each person's response is unique (Dubovsky 1981).

When Ann's doctor (see chapter 5) told her to "avoid stress," she thought he was out of his mind. She was a single, working mother. She had too much to do to be sick, she thought. It would be wonderful if she could just sit home and take it easy, but it wasn't an option. Ann wondered whether all the doctor's patients were happily married and independently wealthy, and he just did not understand what she was up against. Ann assumed she had no choice but to carry on, and struggled with her family, work, and her illness until she could go no further and reached a state of collapse.

Ten years later, Ann understood the words "avoid stress" differ-ently. She understood that her body could withstand only so much before she would suffer the consequences. Her doctor had been try-ing to warn her that her body would only stretch so far and no more. Ann had wanted her body to do more than it was capable of doing. Her illness forced her to learn and accept the limits of her body.

Stress and Your Illness

Living with a chronic illness causes stress, as anyone who has ever had one knows only too well. People who live with Sjögren's syndrome have many stress-related experiences not shared by the general population. These include: dealing with the uncertainty of what will happen next, fear of abandonment, changes in self-esteem and sense of self, isolation, the inability to live as you lived before, anxiety, depression, financial worries, shifting goals and dreams, and the omnipresent encounters with the medical establishment. Sjögren's syndrome can make life a stress-related minefield.

Offsetting Stress

What can you do to offset stress? Remember, stress is universal. What matters is how you perceive it, deal with it, and what you do with it. You can make attempts to limit it, but life without any kind of stress is probably impossible, or close to it. In order to offset stress:

* Find support, both emotional help and instrumental or practical help. Both kinds of support appear to mitigate stress.

* Meet stress head-on. You will be less stressed when you have the feeling that you can exercise some control in a situation, even if you can never have complete control.

* Decide what your limits are, what you can and cannot do. This may be difficult and take time, but it makes a difference if you feel that you are working on the problem.

* Have fun and laugh, even if the effects are only temporary. Fun and laughter counteract stress.

* Treat depression and anxiety.

* Be flexible. Illness makes some people want to seek refuge in the familiar, but that may not give them what they need. Make a deliberate effort, when you can, to step out of the box.

* Exercise to whatever extent is possible. Get out and walk if you can, or swim, or do whatever makes you feel better. If your insurance will pay for it, exercise under the supervision of a physical therapist.

* If it's a bad day, indulge yourself in something, even if it means turning off the phone and taking a bath.

* Eat well.

* Sleep as well as you can.

* Meditate. Faith, prayer, massage, yoga, and many other activities help release and reduce stress. There are many hospital-based stress reduction programs. See if one is offered in your community.

Remember that small changes do add up. Stress is not necessarily the result of large life dramas. It is the composite of small things, especially when compounded by illness. Not everything on this list is appropriate for everyone. You have to figure out what is right for you and what you are both willing and able to do.

Attitude and Emotion

Considerable evidence suggests we may be able to use our minds to influence our bodies. While attitude *may* influence outcome, an exacerbation or new development does not indicate failure. There is no correct attitude or set of emotions that you should have with regard to your illness. The goal is to live the best life you can and to minimize the physical and psychological factors that get in the way. There are many people with wonderful attitudes who do everything right, and still become very sick.

We do not believe that illness is the result of anyone's failure to deal with the world in an effective manner. We do, however, think that you can make a deliberate effort to make your life better and can work to reduce the harmful effects of stress. If stress does make you sick, then finding antidotes that both relieve and release stress may help to make you well; at minimum, it will enable you to better deal with your illness.

Norman Cousins (1979) wrote about his own experience. In 1964, Cousins was diagnosed with ankylosing spondylitis, a crippling and progressive connective tissue disease from which he was given a one in five hundred chance of recovery. Cousins decided that with the unfavorable odds given to him by the medical profession, he would have to do something to improve his chances. In consultation with his physician, he devised a treatment that included massive doses of vitamin C and watching *Candid Camera* and Marx Brothers films. He discovered that the comic relief helped him sleep and found that his pain began to diminish. He steadily improved over a period of years.

Cousins is the first to say he doesn't know why he got better. He writes eloquently about the placebo effect and the possibility that he might have improved without either the vitamin C or the laughter. He remains convinced, however, that it was his refusal to passively accept his fate and his belief that he could do something that would positively affect his condition, along with the full cooperation of his doctors, that enabled him to get well.

Emotions and the "Illness-Prone Personality"

There is a large and often contradictory literature on the relationship between (a) stress and the development of disease and (b) the impact of stress on recovery or intensification of illness. We approach this literature with a critical eye, but feel that it is important to include in this discussion.

It seems highly likely that the mind-body dichotomy is an artificial one. Prolonged stress sets off a series of physiological changes that affect different organ systems in different ways, especially where there is a pre-existing constitutional or congenital weakness or set of weaknesses. One group of researchers describes it well when they say, "Personality styles or mental states do not cause disease so much as they act as a risk factor that, when combined with other risk factors, increases vulnerability" (Hafen et al. 1996, 100).

The way in which a person reacts to stress impacts his or her quality of life. There is little controversy about this, as there is little controversy about the fact that some people are able to tolerate remarkable amounts of stress with no illness-related consequences. What is questionable is whether any specific personality type, traits, or emotions contribute to the development of autoimmune diseases.

Since the 1940s many studies have argued a link between certain personality characteristics and the development of disease. For those interested in a more complete discussion, we refer the reader to *Mind/Body Health* (Hafen et al. 1996). These authors offer a discussion of the researchers who feel that there is a generic disease-prone personality. According to this research, people with certain personality traits are likely to develop disease. To balance the discussion, they cite a discussion of the work of Dr. Barrie Cassileth and her colleagues (1985) who studied advanced cancer patients and found no correlation between attitude (either positive or negative) and survival.

There are numerous studies about emotions, emotional states, personality, and cancer, including some about leukemia and lymphoma. Greene (1966), studied men and women with leukemia and lymphoma and found that although there was no common personality type among the participants, the disease appeared to have developed at a time when the individuals studied had experienced a significant personal loss of an important figure, such as a wife or mother.

In an earlier study, Greene and his colleagues suggested that this loss of support might be a precipitating factor in the development of disease, although they do say that they considered it only one factor that might have caused disease to develop (Greene, Young, and Swisher 1956).

How should these studies be interpreted? Very carefully, in our opinion. Many of these early studies seem too simplistic and appear to place blame. Some have been outdated by recent medical discoveries that lead to increased understanding of the interaction between emotions and the immune system. Others have simply been outdated by advances in science and technology. More sophisticated research will increase our understanding of the biological basis of the mind-body interaction.

If we believe in the mind-body connection, we should use it to our advantage. We will never have complete control of our lives, but each of us can take a proactive position and assume responsibility for our well-being. Attitudes towards control tend to develop early in life, but in general, most of us do better when we feel we can influence the way we interact with the world. We can be proactive in a variety of ways: getting enough support, taking steps to reduce and relieve stress, and keeping ourselves as well as possible with the help of our doctors, family, and friends.

8

Family and Friends

It's difficult to know what to say when someone asks, "How are you?" Should you say "I'm fine" when you're not? Or should you tell the person how you really feel? Telling someone how you feel means acknowledging your illness. Saying you're fine when you're not fits the rhetorical nature of the question. When you have Sjögren's syndrome, the answer to this question can be a dilemma.

Having an illness affects not only the person with the disease, but that person's partner, family, friends, and colleagues. It factors into all of your relationships and into many of your decisions about relationships.

The way you react influences the way others react to you. In return, their response influences the way that you are able to cope. Positive relationships help; negative ones hurt. Even after years of living with Sjögren's, it hurts when family and friends insinuate that you did something to bring it on yourself or when they fail to realize that there is anything wrong with you.

Real Life versus the Movies

Some people believe that illness is inherently ennobling. Illness does not automatically bring on a series of epiphanies or make you wise, nor does it make you more sympathetic. Hollywood versions of illness make the arrogant humble and bring families together.

In real life, illness creates misunderstandings and disrupts relationships as much as it brings people closer together. For some people, it is just one more thing that happens in life and is accepted as such, but living with chronic illness can be difficult, even draining. Let us take a look at three different scenarios.

Denial

Family and friends don't know what to say or how to act, so they pretend it just isn't happening. Sometimes it is too painful for them to acknowledge the wide-reaching ramifications of your having Sjögren's. They want you to be well. You look healthy, therefore you are. Alternatively, you may be in denial. Family and friends are aware something is wrong, but they aren't sure what. They look for signs and symptoms and may misinterpret perfectly normal occurrences as illness-related behavior. Illness is easiest to deny when it is invisible, or when the signs are so vague that they might mean anything.

Too Much Detail

In this scenario, when an inquiry is made, you let the person who is asking know the detailed status of the disease. When you do this, you run the risk of telling the inquirer more than he or she wants to hear. You also risk defining yourself in terms of your illness. In turn, the person may tell you about her most recent episode of the flu, the one that dragged on for weeks, or his back problems, varicose veins, and so on. She or he may claim to know just how you feel. You end up feeling that this person doesn't understand at all or that you are the sum of your symptoms. It can be frustrating when this happens.

Report from the Middle Ground

An inquiry about your health is answered on the basis of your knowledge of the person asking the question. You answer some people in detail and tell others you are fine. It takes time to sort this out and you may make some mistakes along the way. Fortunately, "How are you?" is a question asked often enough that any errors can be corrected the next time the question is asked.

Deirdre's Story

Some of the most eloquent comments on relationships with family and friends have come from people who have lived with Sjögren's syndrome. When Deirdre was asked about how her lupus and Sjögren's affected her relationship with her husband, she offered the following answer:

> [My husband] did well to keep positive over the years, but recently he has had to admit to himself that I am not going to get better and may get worse. I have found the best way to approach this is to keep my self-respect in all situations, and maintain a level of honesty and openness in our relationship. Even at my worst, I do expect respect from others. Sometimes I dribble because of loss of feeling in my face, and sometimes much worse, but I am not these things. I am something more and believe this passionately. Here are some of my basic principles:
>
> I am the way I am and cannot change that. My limitations do not mean I am restricted, but they act as the kicking-off point for all I can do. It is a way of thinking. I had a fulfilling career, but those days are gone and will never come back. All of my academic and career achievements have been replaced by an understanding of how life itself is of the utmost importance, as are family and friends. I am still needed and look for ways I can give to others. I do not want a martyr for a partner. [My husband] is entitled to move on if what he wants from life is a fit wife. As it happens, he has discovered depths in our relationship that he would not have seen had I had full health. I think we are happier now than ever before, but we work at it.
>
> Looking back, I find one of my greatest pleasures is losing some of my friends because of my illness. The ones that are left are very special. I have chosen my new friends very carefully.

Although she does not have good health, Deirdre is blessed with a healthy attitude, one she has worked hard to achieve. Others are not so fortunate. The onset of an illness changes relationships. As one woman said about her relationship with her husband, "My illness changed the nature of our agreement. I was supposed to work. Now he has full responsibility for our financial situation, and I feel that I am less than an equal partner. For a long time, he was very angry about this, and sometimes he still is. We have had our ups and downs, but we have finally worked out a way to live. Another man might have left. We have found ways to be together."

Dealing with Chronic Illness

"Are you better yet? Are you getting well?" are also difficult questions to answer. You might feel better than the last time you saw the person, or you might feel better than you were a month ago, but you don't feel the way you did before you got sick. It can be difficult to make family and friends understand that this disease will not disappear. As a woman named Gayle said, "How do you make others accept what you have had to accept?"

She also pointed out that you can be lonely even with a large family:

> I've tried hard to educate my family about Sjögren's
> syndrome, polymyalgia, and diabetes. I have all three.
> I live twenty-five miles from my mother, where most family
> get-togethers are held. I have a big family—ten brothers
> and sisters. I feel blessed if I feel good enough to visit my
> mother for a few hours, but I am rarely well enough to
> attend family functions. My family just keeps after me to
> do this and do that, and I just want to crawl in a hole
> somewhere and hide. I want to see all of them too and
> I am often lonely. I stay in touch via the phone and e-mail.
> Most of the time, I am not able to drive more than a few
> miles safely. My family and friends often ask the question,
> "Are you getting well?

Janice answered that question this way:

> I used to rack my brain and worry to no end about
> trying to educate my family about my health. I tried giving
> them pamphlets to read, tried telling them, etc. I've had

Sjögren's for close to twenty years now and finally gave
up explaining. Certain friends don't "get it" and have closed
their minds to even trying. I don't even think about them
anymore. Certain family members are the same way, but
I have an "it's their loss" attitude now.

Tell your family and friends, "No, there's no cure for
Sjögren's syndrome and I'm not getting well. What I am
doing is taking care of myself. This means that I'd love to
spend more time with you, but cannot drive safely to do
so. I have to rest each and every day. I cannot do what
I used to be able to do. I'd love to spend time with you
for all the family events, but I'm not well enough to do so."

Ask them to come visit with you and bring lunch or
whatever. If you have to put it in writing (which sometimes
makes it easier), then write letters. Tell them you are not
making this up and you want to be like you used to be,
but that was then and this is now, and you're doing
whatever you can to accept it and you hope that they
learn to do so too. Ask for dialogue, discussion, questions.
Ask family members and friends to go with you to doctor's
appointments. Most of all, do whatever is necessary to
move forward. And if they cannot accept it, do whatever is
necessary for you to accept yourself now and in the future.

Nancy, another woman with Sjögren's, found a way to answer
questions about getting well with the help of her rheumatologist. He
advised her to tell them: "No, I am not well, just gratefully *alive.*"
Then, he advised her to add, "And you?"

On the other hand, some people prefer to say very little. Here
is how a woman named Susan copes with these questions:

I think many of us have struggled with this. I believe I lost
several friends in the early years discussing my illness too
much (or at all). You might say, "Well, who needs them?"
but in truth, we all do. I have since adopted an "if you
can't make it, fake it" attitude. . . . Whenever someone asks,
I almost always say. "I'm doing really well," even if I'm
not. You have to remember that "How are you?" is a
rhetorical question, anyway. Even when someone specifically
asks about my illness, I usually give the same answer. . . .
I try to avoid providing a medical excuse if possible.

People tend to be suspicious of them, even when they are completely justified. I am determined to be doing really well, regardless of what evidence there is to the contrary. I know I'm happier (and I believe more functional) with that attitude, and goodness knows everyone around me is too.

There are no right or wrong answers about how to approach your family and friends. Each person must find a way to deal with these questions and all that they imply. Some choose to answer rhetorically, while others provide an explanation of how they feel and what is happening. Some people do both, making a decision about how to answer each time a question is asked. Some people never really make a decision at all. They intuitively know what to do when the situation arises.

Attitudes Can Improve over Time

Family and friends may become more accepting over time as it becomes clear to them what having Sjögren's syndrome really means. Time allows you to clarify what you need from your relationships and to learn how to make changes in your relationships with family and friends. Pat wrote the following:

> I discovered that [family and friends'] minimization and denial of my lack of functioning was an effort not to see me suffering. The thing that helped best with my mother was to take her to a lecture on Sjögren's, given by a rheumatologist. She came out of there horrified and asked me, "Do you have all those symptoms at once?" At that moment she understood the extent of the symptoms. . . . A few graphic photographs of untreated Sjögren's patients with parotids so large you could barely see the ears helped also.
>
>   Now when I tell my family I can't manage to go to two events in one day, they accept it and ask if I'm up to whatever they want to do. . . . I pay the price if I push myself beyond my limits or go to some environment that aggravates my symptoms with drier eyes or more fatigue. I've had to say "no" many times or modify or limit my participation. With my family, I emphasize the need to plan

ahead so I can pace myself. . . . For example, I can't vacuum my house, then sit for three hours in a restaurant . . . so I have to plan to spread out the "endurance activities."

All this is a hard lesson, especially for women who have been brought up to defer to others. Part of accepting your limitations is being able to ask for help, and that's not easy for those who have been brought up to value competence and independence. You need clear limits both for yourself and for others. If you are unaccustomed to being assertive, it may seem strange or even aggressive at first, but it becomes more comfortable with practice.

JoAnn wrote about the changes in her family:

My mother is doing a lot better through a concentrated effort to read the articles that I send her. She is a retired nurse (and dental hygienist) so had some science background that makes translating medical reports and articles easier for her to do than for some other family members. I think her first reaction was denial, because I've been the oldest child that she could always count on for support and any help that was necessary. Now I'm in worse shape than she is, and it was upsetting for her to think about. When she asks how I'm doing, I feel free to tell her whether I'm better than last week or not as good. It's nice to have that open communication with her now.

My sister, also a nurse, doesn't ask me specific questions, but rather asks how I'm feeling that week. My youngest brother, a physician, was most helpful in getting some referrals for me early in my diagnosis phase, but can't seem to come to grips with the facts of this illness, and I rarely hear from him now. The other brother is very supportive, mostly via e-mail since he lives several thousand miles away. His . . . wife has fibromyalgia, so he has had some "sensitivity training" on the realities of autoimmune disease.

Attitudes Can Get Worse

Each of us wants to think that the people we love and care for will stick with us through whatever comes along, but chronic illness creates changes that some relationships are not able to accommodate. It is particularly painful to lose a friend or to lose touch with a family member at a time when you need people. It is not only disappointing when this happens, it can feel like such a betrayal. Carol, a psychologist with Sjögren's who is single, described her experiences:

> In my family, my sisters have been supportive because they too have autoimmune illnesses. My nieces also understand. My parents have a harder time. My mom feels guilty, as if somehow she is to blame because her three daughters are all sick. My dad has a tough-guy attitude, thinking that we should be able to work. As for my friends, I found out who my real friends are—the ones who stuck by me despite my being sick. But I think that even the ones who stuck by me have a difficult time understanding how I feel. The ones that truly understand are the new friends I have made who are also ill.

Janice, who is happily married, comments on how difficult it can be to find new friends when energy is so limited. She has learned to deal with people who are not supportive:

> Being with friends is the one thing I don't do much any more. And I think it has caused a tremendous shift in my emotional well-being. Inasmuch as I'm extremely gregarious, when you don't get together with friends, you get out of the habit of being gregarious. The exhaustion and pain make you not want to do anything. Once you're not doing much of anything, you don't want to get together because you've been away from that side of yourself for so long that it doesn't feel natural. It's not healthy at all.

She has had to deal with negative responses from family and friends. About these, she says: "I honestly do not need people in my life who put me down. Friends, family, or whoever, it doesn't matter. I have enough to deal with, and the negativity is not something I want to listen to."

It is worth noting that many people lose friends and make new ones over the course of a long illness. Friendships shift throughout life. They change with marriage, divorce, moves, changes in financial status, parenthood, as well as changes in health, but losing a friend because of health-related changes seems to involve a particular feeling of vulnerability. The resolve to not tolerate unsupportive relationships that Janice has achieved is often hard-won. As one woman with Sjögren's said, "I am still struggling with the acceptance of my diseases. . . . The hardest part is my immediate family. My husband doesn't have a clue as to my feelings and needs. . . . I guess in a way, I am not who I was and he doesn't want the new me."

The problem with illness is that many of us don't want this "new me" either, but we don't have a choice. As many of these women have said, once they accepted that the reality of their lives had changed, they were able to accept the changes in relationships with family and friends and move on. The friends that remain are the ones who fulfill the true definition of friendship.

You may encounter people who imply, directly or indirectly, that you did something to bring this on yourself. If only you had lived better, not eaten so many sweets, taken better care of yourself, you would not have this disease. Blaming can be a defense. It implies that you did something wrong. It also implies that if the other person were in your situation, he or she would be able to handle it better. Blaming you enables the other person to emotionally protect himself or herself from your experience. From this perspective, you got sick because you were flawed. You stay sick because you don't handle it as well as this other person would.

It Takes a Village

When you are sick, it can be difficult to maintain relationships with friends. On the other hand, it's probably never been more important. The larger the circle of support, the better. Research shows that good friends help offset the effects of stress (Hafen et al. 1996).

Ellen Goodman and Patricia O'Brien write about their long-term friendship in a book called *I Know Just What You Mean* (2000). They describe a woman, a competent, divorced professional in her fifties, who had a head-on collision with her worst fear, a catastrophic illness. After she was diagnosed with breast cancer, one friend realized that despite the matter-of-fact way she was coping, she felt alone and vulnerable underneath. When this woman was alone after a bone marrow transplant, her friend organized thirty women, each of whom would take one day and would ask what she needed. They never left her alone during her convalescence. Some included their husbands in this circle of care and caring. One or two people would have been burdened with so much responsibility, but thirty women with busy lives of their own managed just fine. When she recovered, the woman who had been the object of so much caring formed an organization to provide legal support to poor women with cancer. Such generous acts of kindness are often passed along to others in some different but equally important way.

Family Ties

Positive relationships enable a fighting spirit. Janice, whose illness doesn't permit her much energy to develop friendships, has an extremely strong relationship with her spouse. When asked to describe the effect Sjögren's syndrome has had, Janice replied:

> My husband and I have the most terrific relationship and it's gotten even stronger now than I ever thought possible. One might think that it's inevitable that a marriage/ relationship won't work when one of the partners is chronically ill, but that is not the case for us.
>
> I've had Sjögren's syndrome a whole lot longer than I've known my husband. I told him about it on our second date. Back then, I wasn't very sick, but I had read about what may or may not come with this illness and I wanted to see how he would react to me knowing that I may have serious health problems later on. Plus I didn't want to invest a lot in the relationship had he not been able to handle it. Lucky for me, he and I have been happily married since 1995.
>
> I feel that the key to any successful relationship is to consider it a partnership. My husband and I talk about everything. . . . We were like this before we got married and it's continued to this day. When we said our marriage vows, the part about sickness and health took on a different meaning than perhaps it does for people who aren't in our shoes. Each and every time I get a new diagnosis or a new health problem, my husband tells me that "we'll deal with it and we are a team" and he'll take me any way he can, whether or not I'm ill. And he really means the "we" part.
>
> I am always so surprised and astounded when I read that some spouses leave because the person with the illness

isn't how they were when they got married. I mean, how immature and stupid is that? Everyone is going to age, and with age there are health problems. In my case, my health problems came before I got old.

Janice and her husband, Victor, have a wonderful attitude and are able to communicate effectively. They recognize and accept the reality of Janice's illness. When something happens, Janice feels that Victor will be there for her and they will face whatever problems there are together. No doubt there are many couples who feel this way, but there are others who don't. We could not find any statistics on the incidence of divorce among couples where one spouse has Sjögren's syndrome, but there is little doubt that a chronic illness can put a great deal of stress on a marriage. If the marriage is already stressed and the relationship is brittle, an illness may be the last straw. The well spouse may feel burdened by having too much to do, and disappointed that whatever expectations he or she had are not being met. The illness may cause a change in financial status or may require that a couple hire additional help for household tasks or child care.

On the positive side, families are able to buffer stress and fill in when a person is unable to do something because of illness. A mother's sister attends a child's baseball game, picks up a child at a friend's house, makes dinner, and does the shopping. A brother comes over to help with some carpentry or work in the garden. A cousin trims the hedges. An uncle provides financial help during a difficult time. Unable to work, a daughter moves back home with parents or moves in with a sibling. A family provides love and support because they are family; no other reason is necessary. A strong family makes a person feel that they are loved, cared for, valued, and esteemed, and provides a sense of belonging (Hafen et al. 1996). An extended family widens this circle and provides a feeling of being part of a clan and a community. While it is possible to be lonely in the midst of a large family, families provide a sense of connectedness that helps ward off loneliness and isolation.

Sex and Intimacy

Maintaining a sexual relationship is difficult when you don't feel well, live with pain, and lack energy. Some women may experience a diminution of their sexual drive after menopause, while others find it a time of increased sexual freedom. Sex, or the lack of it, can become another problem, compounding others in a relationship. The well spouse or partner may want sex, but doesn't wish to initiate it, because he knows you would rather go to sleep. He also may not wish to initiate it for fear of being refused. Lack of communication adds to the problem.

Communication is at the heart of sexual intimacy. A couple needs to communicate their likes and dislikes in order to achieve mutual pleasure. When a chronic illness emerges, the feelings of both partners may be reflected through their sexuality. If the person with the disease feels unable to talk to their partner about what is going on inside, it is very likely that this lack of communication will be reflected in their lovemaking. If one partner feels sick and stressed, he or she may not feel like making love. Sometimes people do not like their bodies or feel that they are not as attractive as they were before they got sick. Sex that is a chore will only build further resentment, but a good sexual relationship can carry a couple through some difficult times. Intimacy on one level fosters intimacy on other levels as well.

Sex for women with Sjögren's syndrome may be painful if vaginal dryness is severe. Dryness also increases naturally after menopause. Some women may find this aspect of the disease difficult to talk about, but it is important that your partner understand how you feel. This can be especially difficult in a new sexual relationship, when you are not quite ready to reveal everything about living with Sjögren's. In this case, a little planning is useful. Find out which over-the-counter lubricant works for you. If none of them do, ask your gynecologist for help. People who do not want to take hormone replacement may find relief from vaginal dryness with estrogen used vaginally. Build a relationship slowly. Even if it is in general terms, talk about the ways that Sjögren's affects your life.

If you want to change a long-standing sexual pattern, it helps to be frank. Perhaps your partner is reluctant to initiate sex because he is afraid you are not feeling well. In fact, you don't feel well, but the fact that he doesn't initiate it makes you feel unwanted and afraid that he doesn't want you anymore because of your illness. Let your partner know that you would like to have sex, just not now. Let him know that you will tell him when you feel up to it, so he doesn't have to guess and get it wrong.

Innovative partners will understand that even if you are too tired for intercourse, a massage or tender touching may take on new meaning. Good communication will let your partner know that even if you are too tired for sex, you still want to be touched or held. Or, you may be too tired at night, but feel better about having sex in the morning.

Pregnancy Issues

In addition to medical considerations of pregnancy in Sjögren's syndrome (see chapter 4), you should consider how you will manage taking care of your baby.

* Do you feel able to care for an infant?

* Have you and your partner discussed how the two of you will care for a child?

* If you have other children or you work, are you able to juggle multiple (and sometimes conflicting) responsibilities?

* Is your partner willing and able to be available if you need extra help? If this is not possible, is additional help available if you need it?

Daily Life

Having Sjögren's syndrome can change one thing or everything in your daily life. It can change where you live, what you do, and who you spend time with. It can necessitate moving to a different kind of house, hiring help, letting things go, or asking other family members to do things that you are not able to do. If one person has to cut back or stop working, two incomes become one and the medical bills increase. There can be a prolonged period of adjustment.

Adapting to these changes takes time. It's too much to ask, either of yourself or your partner and family members, to do all at once. Make changes slowly. Try to explain to the people you love that although you look well, you cannot do what you used to do. If they are able to understand this, go one step further. Explain that these unwanted changes are hard to make. They reflect not just changes in the way you live your life, but also in your plans, hopes, and dreams. Giving up hopes and dreams can be every bit as painful and difficult as the reality of having to adjust to living on one salary instead of two.

Unfortunately, even after years, friends and family may react adversely if you express anger or dismay when you don't feel well. Once they accept the fact that you have an illness, and see you accepting the fact that you have an illness, they sometimes forget that it is a daily struggle to live with an illness that doesn't go away.

The Well Spouse

The burden of a chronic illness is shared by the well spouse. The well spouse accommodates, fills in, changes plans, or goes alone when his or her spouse isn't able to do something, and deals with emergencies as they arise. Some people can do this as a matter of course; others are not so good-natured. Sometimes the well spouse observes and recognizes changes even before the person with the illness does. In a less pleasant scenario, some partners hardly understand what is going on at all.

Monica has been married for more than twenty-five years to Jerry, who was diagnosed three years ago with lupus. They have one son, eighteen and a senior in high school. At first, Monica told us, it was difficult to focus on Jerry's illness, because so much else was happening in their lives at the same time. He had been in a car accident, her father had died, and her mother was terminally ill. Jerry had been losing weight, but was diagnosed after he developed a deep vein thrombosis. Although Jerry has continued to work, Monica notes that he is often tired and in pain.

Monica said a number of things made it easier for her to accept her husband's illness. She works, and has always maintained a measure of independence, with both family and friends. She has a friend with fibromyalgia, and gets together with this friend regularly. As a result of their discussions, she feels better able to understand her husband and his illness. The fact that Jerry continues to work full time has also made things easier. He sometimes works from home and will be eligible for retirement at age fifty-five. At one point, they were afraid he would lose his job. Because his concentration is sometimes impaired, Monica feared that he would not be able to find other work, but luckily his job has remained stable.

Monica will also be eligible for retirement at fifty-five, but knows she will have to work longer if Jerry retires early. She feels fortunate that they both have adequate pensions and health benefits. She is grateful that Jerry's illness did not develop until their son was a teenager, because her husband has always been an extremely active father and it would have been difficult for him not to be an active participant in his son's life. She feels that so far his illness has had relatively little impact on their son, who, as a teenager, has his own concerns.

Jerry comes from a large family, but they are not close. Monica feels that his mother has had a difficult time facing the reality of her son's illness. "She wouldn't call us," she said, "because she didn't want to hear about his not feeling well." Only one of his five siblings stays in touch on a regular basis. She wishes his siblings lived nearby, so they could see what Jerry goes through. She and Jerry both exercise frequently, and she believes that this has helped ward off anxiety and depression. She sums it up by saying, "I guess in life there are no guarantees."

Monica's easygoing temperament has been advantageous in dealing with her husband's illness. She and Jerry have been together a long time, and she is usually able to take things as they come. In addition, she feels that she has an independent life and would continue her activities if Jerry were to become increasingly disabled. They are not affluent but have financial security. Their son is about to go off on his own, and this too is an important factor.

Not everyone is able to take such things in stride. A chronic illness engenders frustration, anger and resentment. Deirdre, the woman who spoke so eloquently about living with her illness, has also written about feeling that her husband was not supportive enough during a recent medical crisis. Once they discussed it, it turned out that he was angry because he could do so little for her at a time when the doctors were not responsive. What she felt was his anger.

A spouse may be good at providing one kind of support, but not another. A husband may be very good at organizing things so that life proceeds smoothly but is unresponsive to his wife's emotional needs, or the opposite may be true. It is probably never a good idea to have all your support come from one person; and remember that even the most supportive spouse sometimes needs a break, or has a bad day and is unresponsive. It is also a good idea for a well spouse to have some outside interests and be able to pursue them on a regular basis.

A Caretaker's Role

Is the well spouse a caretaker? According to Gregg Piburn, a man whose wife, Sherrie, developed fibromyalgia, he became one. He wrote about his experiences in a book published by the Arthritis Foundation, entitled *Beyond Chaos* (1999). When Sherrie went from being a very healthy and athletic mother of two children (they adopted a third after she became sick), Gregg found that the easy life he expected to have had become difficult. His initial tendency was to treat his wife like a china doll and assume responsibility for almost everything. In his book, he chronicles why this stance failed and how, both as a couple and as a family, they came to terms with living with illness.

This book contains some thought-provoking ideas. It is a resource for those with a chronic illness and their families. Gregg does not sugarcoat his experiences. He talks about how he coped (sometimes not so well), in terms that everyone can understand. The book contains good advice for husbands about accompanying wives to doctor's appointments, and it makes a plea for honesty in the relationship. He speaks frankly about sex and about the difficulties of being a caretaker.

He points out that caretakers are also vulnerable. Gregg tried to maintain a stoic facade. He says he was afraid to be afraid. He wondered what his wife would think of him, whether she would respect and love him, but he ultimately concluded that the ability to share feelings gives a couple the necessary freedom to go on with life.

Family Responsibilities

Gregg Piburn learned lessons that many women know from experience. As we age, it is not unusual to find ourselves caught between caring for elderly parents and children at home. Children get sick, break bones, and require surgery. Parents age and need help with medical problems, driving, and getting to doctor's appointments. Spouses lose jobs, and a family must relocate. Whether it is a spouse, parent, or child, it is difficult to assume responsibility for someone else when you can barely take care of yourself. The reality is that this happens often and when it does, the juggling of multiple and often conflicting roles is exhausting and stressful.

It is especially difficult to make decisions about how much you can do if you have a child or a parent with a serious and chronic illness. It helps if other people share the responsibilities, but if you are the primary caretaker, try to pace yourself for the long haul as best you can, delegate or let unessential things go, and figure out what you must do, what you can do, and what you can leave undone.

There's a saying, "Life is what happens while you're making other plans." It doesn't stop because you have Sjögren's or any other illness. Each of us makes decisions based on what we are capable of doing. One of the lessons learned, perhaps sooner rather than later in the presence of significant medical problems, is that no one is perfect and most people do the best they can in an imperfect world. Illness can make us feel both humble and appreciative, both for the efforts we make and for the efforts made by others. There may not be an ideal way of dealing with a particular problem. Some problems are just too big, and we deal with them as best we can. If we have done our best, then we have done what we are capable of doing. It may not be possible to meet other people's expectations. Only you know what you are capable of doing.

You may feel especially guilty about the things you can't do with your children. You may worry that time lost to illness takes away your effectiveness as a parent. It is hard not to be able to attend a ball game or soccer practice, or not be able to do some long-awaited activity with your child. Keep the lines of communication open. If you can't do something, make sure your child knows it's not his or her fault. Let them know that even if you don't feel well, you are still available to them emotionally. They can still tell you about their day, share worries and concerns, and make plans for some other time. Perhaps they will learn what it means to be flexible. Remember that they love you for who you are, not for what you can do.

Effects on Children

Illness in a parent affects a child in many of the same ways that it affects the parent. Depending on their age, children may feel guilty, angry, stressed, anxious, afraid, or depressed. Very young children cannot express their feelings in words, and even older children may have a hard time doing so. They know you are sick and do not want to add any additional stress. Instead, they may act out or isolate themselves. Talk with your children about what is happening on a level they can understand. Do not pretend that everything is fine when it isn't. Children usually know when someone is not telling them the truth, and that may make them even more fearful. If you are worried about something, tell your children you are worried. You need not share all the details, but you can share the feeling of uncertainty or concern. Acknowledging what they observe will validate the reality of their perceptions.

Stressed Families

Without reference to illness, *Mind/Body Health* (Hafen et al. 1996) lists the top stress factors for families today as: "Economics, finances and budgeting, children's behavior, discipline and sibling fighting, insufficient couple time, lack of shared responsibility in the family, (difficulty) communicating with children, insufficient personal time, guilt for not accomplishing more, poor spousal relationships, insufficient family play time, overscheduled family calendar" (342).

To these everyday stresses, dealing with Sjögren's can add:

* too many doctor's appointments

* too much time lost to not feeling well

* lost income and increased financial pressure

* a well spouse who feels stressed and burdened

* an unwell spouse who feels stressed and burdened

* children who feel burdened by their parents' burdens

* inability to do the things that used to give pleasure and relieve stress

* stoicism, or not wishing to share feelings with other family members for fear of making things worse

* anger and depression that result from the above

When you need to take on a prolonged and serious caretaking role and you have Sjögren's syndrome, you may feel the added stress of:

* too many conflicting roles

* too little energy

* risk of illness due to prolonged stressful conditions
* additional financial expenditures
* exhaustion, anger, and depression from all of the above

Divorce and Remarriage

It would be incorrect to think that it is always the well spouse who leaves a marriage because they cannot deal with their partner's illness. Any life crisis can be an opportunity to sort out what is really meaningful and important in life. Illness is no exception. Marriages fail because of chronic illness, especially when the illness is combined with an already stressed marriage. A well spouse may leave if they are unable to deal with their partner's illness, but other factors, such as poor communication or a troubled history, are likely to be just as important when the marriage dissolves. A woman with a long history of being unhappy in a marriage may decide to leave after illness is diagnosed.

Like anyone else, people with Sjögren's syndrome marry and marry again after divorce. As Janice said, the phrase "in sickness and in health" has a different meaning when one or both spouses have chronic health problems. It may be a blessing to meet someone after the illness has already made its debut, so that you can be frank about what it means to you to have it.

Get to know someone well enough so that he or she knows you, and you know how he or she reacts during emergencies. If you have a fever of 104 and your partner doesn't offer you some water or take you to the doctor or the emergency room, he or she is probably not someone who can adapt to living with a chronic illness. If your partner is someone who cannot be flexible, and who will be angry and disappointed each time you need to change or cancel plans, this person is probably not for you. An important question when evaluating a potential mate is, "Is this person someone with whom I can share my experiences?" If the answer is no, think again before committing yourself.

If You Are Single

Carol, the psychologist who spoke about her family and friends earlier in this chapter, was in her early thirties when her disease began. Now in her forties, she says her limited energy has curtailed her social life, especially her relationships with men:

About being young and single, I don't really feel young.
I can tell you that being sick has limited my social life and
in particular my relationships with men. I have a hard time
believing that a man could be interested in being with me,
given that I am sick. I know there are a few good men out
there who would not care about being with someone who
is ill. But I don't have the energy to look for such a man.

When you are getting to know someone, how and when do
you tell them about your health problems? Various schools of
thought exist. The first says to divulge relatively early in the relationship. That way, it's out in the open, and the other person has the
right to decide whether to continue the relationship. "I have multiple
sclerosis," a friend told the man who had just taken her out to dinner
for the first time. He didn't flinch, and ten years later they were still
living together, but she took a chance and knew it. When he didn't
leave, she felt free to proceed.

The problem with this approach is that if you tell too much too
soon, the other person may not have enough context for the information. The disease becomes too large an issue. Therefore, some
people advise waiting a bit, and divulging slowly, in bits and pieces,
with a chance to evaluate how the other person handles each bit of
information.

Carol speaks frankly when she says that although she knows
there are men out there who would not be turned away by her illness, she knows that there are others who would. When this happens, it hurts. If you are single with Sjögren's, you need to decide
how much energy you want to put into searching for a mate and act
accordingly. Janice, who told her (now) husband about having
Sjögren's on their second date, found out not only that he could
handle the fact that she had it, but that he could be a willing partner,
sharing Sjögren's with her, along with the other aspects of their lives.

Middle-Aged Dating

Dating in middle age and beyond may be easier. Because more
people have health problems of their own as they age, they may be
more accepting of the health problems of others. If it's not health
problems, most people in middle age have something they worry
about. When Arthur met Helen, both were in their mid-fifties. He
had Sjögren's syndrome secondary to very severe rheumatoid

arthritis, which was controlled with high doses of medication that had potentially severe side effects. Although Helen was extremely healthy, she had been married three times before and was afraid that if she told Arthur he would think she was a poor relationship risk. Arthur was limping when he came to their first date and explained his health problems right away. Helen waited until they became involved before telling him about her three previous marriages. The point is that each had something they were uneasy about, and each handled it in a different way. They lived together for almost a decade before they tied the knot last year, both now in their sixties.

It's important to remember that just because one person has a high level of activity, it doesn't mean he or she demands the same in a mate. Someone who likes to hike and bike and scuba dive and mountain climb may not expect their partner to do those things with them, as long as they don't stop them from pursuing the activities they love. Relationships are often based on a common interest, but someone who runs marathons may also play the cello or bridge, or love red wines or antiques, or any variety of things that someone who happens to have Sjögren's may be interested in.

If you want to meet someone, it is essential to get out and socialize. Some people decide just to live their lives, open to the possibility of a relationship. Others take a more deliberate approach. They join activity clubs, go dancing, join political groups, use the Internet, or put an ad in the personals. We know of one couple who met online and who have since lived happily ever after. We know people who sat next to each other on a plane, at a time when neither was looking for a partner. Fate intervened and they met. We do not advocate any particular approach. You have to do whatever feels right for you. Unless you are using one of the computer dating services, you are unlikely to meet someone while sitting at home. Meeting someone requires luck, persistence, and a measure of ingenuity. Decide what you can do, set your own pace, and go!

Living Alone

As increasing numbers of people live alone, there are bound to be more people living alone with a chronic disease. Living alone can be both a blessing and a curse. When you live alone, you can schedule your time according to the way you feel. You don't have to go somewhere because your partner wants to go. On the other hand, when you live alone you are responsible for everything, and just getting everything done takes a lot of energy. There's no one around to pay the bills, do the taxes, go to the cleaners or the bank or the grocery store. If you don't do it, it doesn't get done.

When you live alone, you need to plan in order to have a social life. Planning can be problematic when you don't feel well, or when you can't predict how you are going to feel. It means that if you want to do something on the spur of the moment, there may be no one available to do it with. There may be times when you would do something, if only you didn't have to make a round of phone calls first, or if there was someone to do the driving, or drive at least part of the way to wherever you wanted to go. Living alone means there is no one on hand with whom you can share anxious feelings, but it also means that you do not have to pretend to be anything other than what you are.

Alone and lonely are not synonymous. As Joan, a divorced woman with Sjögren's syndrome said:

> I never felt more alone with my illness than when I was married. Now, if something goes wrong, there can be some difficult moments, but I call a friend or a family member, and we talk and usually I'm all right. Of course, there are few people you can call in the middle of the night, and I've had some anxious nights, nights when I thought the next day would never come, but those have been relatively few in number over the past fifteen years. I've grown used to living alone. I won't say that I like it, but in fact, sometimes I do. Because I live alone, I've had to develop a good support system. I don't think I would have done that had I stayed married. I keep up with as many outside interests as I am able. If I could have had a good marriage, that's what I would have chosen. But I didn't have a good marriage and I haven't met anyone else. I'd rather live alone than in a marriage that was always a disappointment. At least this way, I can be myself.

Surrogate Families

One solution to living alone or far away from your family is to build a surrogate family. Whether you are married or single, it helps to have people with whom you can spend holidays and share child care, people with whom you can go on vacation. They may be neighbors, members of the same church or synagogue, or simply people with whom you develop a friendship over time. Leslie and Elena are good examples of women who have created surrogate families. Leslie is a married woman who lived in Boston for many years before she married when she was almost forty and moved to Maryland.

Because she grew up in New England and lived there until she was thirty-nine, she continues to feel that is where her real friends are. Leslie and her husband have no children, and no family near their present home. Leslie spends a part of each year in their summer home and during those months spends time with her close family and friends. She recently celebrated her fifty-fifth birthday with a party of women, and feels as close to these long-time friends as she does to her own brothers and sisters. Leslie has broadened her definition of family to include her long-standing friendships. Family to her is composed of her family of origin and the family she has created over the years.

Elena emigrated from the Soviet Union almost thirty years ago. She came with her husband and two children. Her parents joined them a few years later. She has since divorced and remarried, and her elder daughter is married with two children of her own. Every Saturday night, eleven or twelve people, both family and friends, gather at Elena's home for dinner and conversation. They are a surrogate family.

Surrogate families do not just happen. They form slowly, over time, because they fill a need. Some may be large and extended groups of friends and family. Others are quite small. What is important is the sense of shared connectedness. These are more than just friendships. These are the people who will take you to the emergency room or meet you there. They are the people with whom you can share both joy and sorrow, the people with whom you can be yourself.

9

Living with
Sjögren's Syndrome

Sjogren's affects people so differently and the extent of the disease usually determines the modifications necessary. This chapter is about maintaining your quality of life with Sjögren's syndrome. People with little pain or fatigue do not have to pace themselves in the way that people with either or both do. Age and stage of life make a difference too. Although the actual symptoms and emotions that accompany a diagnosis of Sjögren's may not vary with age, the demands of life are different at thirty-five than at sixty.

Limitations are difficult when you are juggling multiple roles: parent, worker, spouse, and sometimes the caretaker of aging parents with health problems of their own. It makes a difference if you get sick and your family and friends cannot relate to your experience because you are young. In midlife, when people begin to experience health problems, there is more understanding of what it means to have an illness, even if no one has heard of Sjögren's syndrome.

Listen to Your Body

A healthy body takes you where you want to go. Healthy bodies, even those that have reached middle age and beyond, usually move through the day with ease, prone to some aches and pains now and then, prone to afternoon postprandial fatigue, but resilient just the same. Healthy bodies move through a crowd without bringing home an infection that will take weeks to heal, and a healthy body can push itself when the need arises. One healthy friend of ours noted that she gets tired when she pushes herself too far, but it doesn't take her much time to recover. As we write this, we are in awe of what a healthy body can do, with little tending. Sjögren's can make a young person feel old. A healthy seventy-year-old may be able to do more than a person of thirty-five or forty with Sjögren's, and do it with ease.

Listening to your body means paying attention to things you may not want to hear, such as early warning signs of wear and fatigue. Gains from getting one or two more things done are offset by the penalty for doing them. Getting to know your body becomes an important survival tactic.

We aren't suggesting that you constantly check yourself. There's no need to take your temperature (either literally or figuratively), morning, noon, and night. We mean that you need to get to know your body, and what it can and can't do, in an intimate and personalized way. There are times when life circumstances may require more than your body willingly permits, and at such times, do the best you can and make as many adjustments as you can. If you listen to your body, you will find your baseline. If your Sjögren's is not stable, this becomes more difficult. It may take extra time to adapt to change.

Listening to your body is a two-part proposition. Once you think you have a sense of what you can do, you have to pay attention to it! Think of your body as you would your finances. The credit card bill comes at the end of the month and you have to find a way to pay. So it is with your body. If you push it too far, it will let you know and there will be a price to pay. What you can do may change on a daily basis.

Watching Your Limits

It's easy to say "listen to your body," but what about earning a living, taking care of children, going to school, managing a relationship, or taking care of aged parents? There are serious health consequences for pushing yourself beyond your limits. Here are a few suggestions:

* Make small changes if big ones are not possible. See how your body responds. Small changes do add up.

* Have a contingency plan. Ask yourself what you would do if you couldn't do what you are currently doing. Review and revise this as circumstances change.

* Write down your plan in a notebook and put that book away in a safe place. It's always better to make alternative plans and not use them than it is to have to make important decisions in an emergency.

* Push yourself only when absolutely necessary and for the shortest time possible.

Having Sjögren's necessitates choices that a healthy person doesn't have to make. A woman in her thirties with young children at home told us she was contemplating a job change. She had two job offers. One was more interesting, but it was farther away and would require more travel time. The other was closer to home, but less interesting. She thought she would probably take the one closer to home, because it would enable her to go on working for a longer period of time. Here was one woman, like many, whose career was affected by her illness.

You have to make choices all the time. Some of those choices need to take into account that you have Sjögren's. For example, if you have a choice of health plans at work, take the most comprehensive one that you can afford and that gives you the most choice. It won't be the cheapest. Don't try to save money by overlooking the disability insurance if it is optional. Purchase whatever disability insurance you can. Having a chronic disease is a wake-up call to the fact that unpleasant things do happen, and it pays to take a long view.

Containing Flares

A flare is an exacerbation of symptoms. Joints hurt more, muscles ache, fatigue increases, and there is no other obvious cause. For some people, it is difficult to differentiate a Sjögren's flare from the flu or an infection that produces nonspecific symptoms. Flares may trigger depression, and it is difficult to distinguish between the symptoms of depression and those of a flare. Doctors can have trouble differentiating too, so when you go in and say "I'm feeling worse," they may take some routine lab tests, and if those don't provide any more specific clues, they may adopt a "wait and see what develops" attitude. Once a flare begins, it's difficult to say how long it will last. Some flares last a few days. Others persist for weeks.

Some flares occur after a specific incident. Stress can provoke one, as can viral or bacterial infections and some medical procedures. The infection ends, but sometimes symptoms persist and you continue to feel worse than usual. You may run a low-grade fever.

Fluctuations can also occur within a flare. For a few hours, a part of a day, or even for a day or two, you may feel better. Just as you begin to think it's over, it comes back.

Once a flare begins, it is hard to make adjustments. No matter how limited you are, you probably make plans based on what you expect to be able to do. When you can't do what you expected, you face the consequences of not getting it done, and also your feelings about not being able to do what you had planned.

"Will this ever go away?" is a question frequently asked during a flare. In most cases, the answer is a hopeful "Yes, this too shall pass." First you have to get through it. Learn what you can about your body from the flare. If it occurred after some specific activity, think about ways you might moderate this activity in the future. Remember that sometimes cause and effect isn't so obvious. Before you decide that a vacation with your in-laws caused a flare, think about the full range of factors involved: extra energy getting ready for the trip, the stresses of travel, unfamiliar surroundings, changes in climate, and so on.

Once a flare occurs, simplify. Give in and let your body rest as much as possible. Take time off from work, sleep extra hours, let the housework go, and order take-out or let someone else cook. Don't burden yourself with guilt. Stare at the television if you need to, take a warm bath, read a book. The idea is to get through it as quickly as possible. Flares are always unwelcome guests. Think of them that way and look forward to the day they go home.

Coping with Pain

Pain is part of Sjögren's syndrome for many people. It may be the result of fibromyalgia or it may be part of primary Sjögren's. It may be muscle or joint pain and may be acute and chronic. People with Sjögren's may have a variety of overlapping conditions that cause pain, such as fibromyalgia, arthritis, tendinitis, migraines, or irritable bowel syndrome.

Pain control can be an arduous process. It may take multiple trials of a nonsteroidal anti-inflammatory drug (NSAID) to find one that works. For some people, the side effects may be as bad or almost as bad as the symptom the medication is meant to control. Multiple medication trials may be required, which becomes excruciating to someone who just wants his or her pain to go away. Sometimes it is difficult to keep trying. As author Suzanne Skevington notes, "unless pain sufferers have a reasonable expectation that if they take a particular course of action that will be able to directly control their pain, they are unlikely to attempt it" (Skevington 1995, p144). People who feel that they will ultimately be able to get their pain under control are likely to be more tolerant of the unpleasant side effects than those who fear that they will not be able to control their pain (Skevington 1995). Inadequate pain control may be worse than having no control at all, which makes perseverance all the more important.

Education and behavioral changes are important components of pain control. Self-management courses that combine information about arthritis, exercise and relaxation programs, and information on nutrition and medication use have been found to decrease pain and depression significantly, and the results were sustained over time. Four years after patients had entered a program, their pain was still 20 percent less than at the beginning of treatment (Skevington 1995). The combination of education and behavioral changes appeared to be more effective than either education or behavior change alone.

Chronic pain can lead to an increase in depression, and depression may lead to a decreased ability to cope with chronic pain. In one study, the researchers found that people with inflammatory disease had higher levels of pain after an unpleasant day (Skevington 1995). The same researchers found that people who had high levels of social support were likely to have less pain and depression after something unpleasant occurred, indicating that social support can act as an important buffer.

People with chronic pain may feel increasingly depressed if they sense that other people are withdrawing or do not understand their experience, or fail to appreciate the limitations and restrictions of living with chronic pain. Kleinman (1988) notes that depression that results from chronic pain may actually be the result of demoralization. This is exacerbated if physicians fail to recognize the extent of your pain and don't treat it adequately. It is therefore extremely important to discuss any uncontrolled or poorly controlled pain with your physician and to have the same conversation repeatedly, if necessary.

Coping with Fatigue

Fatigue, in all its textures and nuances, is part of life for many people with Sjögren's. The fatigue that accompanies Sjögren's has been characterized as awful, terrible, bone-tired, bone-weary, toxic, encompassing, poisonous, and noxious. It invades and engulfs, attacks, assaults, inundates, swallows, and entombs. It is a fatigue that makes some people feel as if they are a piece of laundry. They "crumple and fold" like a limp bed sheet or a towel on the floor. In his book on lupus, Robert Phillips says people with lupus (and Sjögren's) feel "as if someone had pulled the plug" (Phillips 2001, 53). We agree with him.

One of the difficult things about Sjögren's-related fatigue is that it comes on so swiftly. You can feel normal in the morning, and as if there were lead weights attached to every limb by noon. The fatigue may be accompanied by an increase in joint or muscle pain. Fatigue can be a constant companion. We have each had the experience of waking up in the morning and feeling that someone had poured molten lead into our bodies overnight. When the fatigue is sudden, it's difficult to continue what you are doing. It's hard to concentrate. In the middle of a meeting or some other activity, we have each become too tired to talk. We have put down writing this manuscript in the middle of a sentence.

It is possible to be incredibly tired and still appear normal. Because pain and fatigue are invisible, most people won't know what you are feeling unless you tell them. When someone knows you well, they learn to pick up subtle signs. "Do you want to go home, Mom?" one of our children said recently after an afternoon of shopping. After so many years, he had learned to recognize when his mother was ready to fold. Mom gratefully handed her grown-up son the car keys.

You may be sensitive to changes in either temperature or barometric pressure, or both. You know that a storm is moving in while the sky remains blue and cloudless. When the temperature shifts dramatically or the barometric pressure rises or falls, you can feel a corresponding wave of fatigue or feel released from fatigue.

Other medical causes of fatigue should be ruled out. Fatigue is a nonspecific symptom that accompanies many different conditions. Among these are diabetes, thyroid conditions, anemia, infection, cancer, and other autoimmune diseases.

Fatigue can be a side effect of medication, but medication can also help alleviate fatigue. A variety of medications that work for pain also help alleviate fatigue: some of the NSAIDs, Plaquenil, and prednisone are examples. Fatigue can result from poor nutrition (because you are too tired to cook or shop) and, paradoxically, from inactivity. Fatigue may also be the result of depression.

Dealing with Dryness

Dryness can affect the quality of your life. You may have very dry eyes, but your mouth is less dry, or vice-versa. You may not be able to get through the day without large amounts of water and eyedrops, or get through the night without waking up to take a drink or put ointment in your eyes. Your eyes may be sensitive to light, and you may avoid driving or riding in cars or walking in the wind because it aggravates already dry eyes. Dryness can restrict the amount of time you are able to spend working at a computer or reading.

Dryness can hit your pocketbook hard, too. Eyedrops, special mouth rinses and toothpastes, and tiny tubes of eye ointment add up to a significant annual expense.

If dryness prevents you from sleeping through the night, make sure the humidity in your home is adequate. There are inexpensive thermometers that measure both temperature and humidity. While forty percent humidity is desirable, in certain parts of the country you are lucky when you can humidify your home to more than 30 percent. Remember that both heat and air-conditioning are drying. Unfortunately, a humidifier or humidification system can be a good source for both mold and bacteria. Whether you have tabletop humidifiers or a built-in system, careful maintenance is essential.

Getting Enough Rest

People with autoimmune diseases need extra rest and often don't get it. You may have trouble falling asleep or staying asleep and wake up feeling as if you haven't slept at all. Extra rest may mean needing to take breaks during the day.

You may not do well with long periods of sustained activity. Whenever possible, try to rest. One friend with Sjögren's divides the day into three periods, morning, afternoon, and evening. If she does something in the morning, and knows that she has plans for the evening, the afternoon is designated as mandatory rest time. If she has to do something in both the morning and afternoon, she is tired by four or five, and needs to rest all evening. When she is not feeling well, she might do something in the morning and rest for the remainder of the day. Another friend prepares dinner early because she needs to rest in the afternoon.

Resting is difficult when you have a job, young children, or both. Sometimes a half hour or forty-five minutes will help. Twenty minutes is better than nothing. Try to carve out some time when you can just sit down and recharge.

How Much Should You Push Yourself?

If you never pushed yourself, life would be devoid of challenge, as well as boring. You may push yourself to do new things, to accomplish something that seems just beyond your reach, or to change from one situation to something else. If you push yourself too often and too far, you pay the price. It's important to achieve the right balance. It's like walking a tightrope. Lean too far to one side, and you compromise what you can do with your life. Lean to the other, and you will find yourself exhausted and in a state of constantly needing to recuperate. How far you should push yourself is therefore exceedingly personal. It relates to what we said earlier about listening to your body. Stay as active as you can without paying too great a price. Sometimes it is necessary to do something that is a challenge. You may be able to do more and go further than you think, but challenge yourself gently.

How Can I Live with This *&^%! Disease?

Living well is still the best revenge. People who are emotionally healthy tend to have traits that enhance their ability to endure despite difficult times. Ornstein and Sobel (1989) say that emotionally healthy people tend to remember their successes more than their failures and assume that their ability to influence events is more than it actually is. Healthy people believe they can take control of a situation and feel hopeful about the future, two important coping mechanisms. They are enhanced by social relationships and tend to have a good support system.

We can hear the protests now—living with a chronic disease makes a person feel out of control, distances them from their healthy friends and family members who have a hard time dealing with their illness, and makes it difficult to hope for the future when it is impossible just to get from one day to the next. The following sections deal with ways to improve life, with or without Sjögren's syndrome.

Find Pleasure

Not all pleasure has to come from large or important moments. Researchers asked whether it was "how positive people felt" versus "how often people felt positive" that was important to happiness and well-being. They found that simple pleasures, more frequently felt, appeared more important than a few large and memorable happy occasions (Ornstein and Sobel 1989). The implications of this are that if you have something that makes you happy, even for a short time, on a daily or frequent basis, you will feel better. Better than what? Well, better in a sense of overall well-being than if you don't have anything that makes you happy. Examples of this can be working in the garden, walking the dog, reading a good book, listening to a wonderful piece of music (or playing it), meeting a friend for coffee, or just talking on the phone with a good friend every day.

It is also important to continue to do things you love to do. You should have something to look forward to and do things you enjoy. Figure out what brings you pleasure and do it as often as you can.

Get Enough Support

Remember, finding enough support can be difficult with a disease like Sjögren's. Support can be emotional or practical, and it's important to remember that not everyone is capable of both.

Emotional support comes from the friend or family member who listens, understands, and is there with a word or a hug that reminds you there is someone in the world you can count on. Practical support is more functional in nature. This kind of support comes from the person who goes to the doctor with you, or drives you someplace that's difficult to get to, or takes your dog for a walk and picks up the cleaning if you can't manage it.

Make a List

In an ideal world, both kinds of support would come from the same person, but in the real world, this may not be the case. Here's what you can do about it:

- List the important people in your life. Think about each person and what qualities he or she possesses.

- Put an E for *emotional,* P for *practical,* or both letters next to each name. Ask each person only for what you think he or she can give. Experience will tell you if you have judged correctly.

- Revise the list periodically. Add new people; delete names if necessary. Adjust your ideas of what friends and family can do to help. Sometimes people surprise you as you get to know them better, in both positive and negative ways.

- Remember that support is a two-way street, and that you can still support others as they support you. Support that is one-directional won't endure over time. In fact, Ornstein

and Sobel (1989) list altruism as one of their "healthy pleasures." Focusing on others keeps you connected, and there
is evidence that your connection to others has the beneficial
effect of buffering stress (Ornstein and Sobel 1989).

Take a task-oriented approach to enlarging your support system. Work at it when you can. For a variety of reasons, it seems to
be more difficult to make good friends as you get older, perhaps
because people are more immersed in and occupied with their own
lives. Sometimes support comes from people who are kind strangers
or acquaintances. You may have numerous false starts before you
make one new friend, but it's important to keep trying, because that
one person may make all the difference.

Support groups are available through the Sjögren's Syndrome
Foundation. Online support and discussion groups are also available. See Resources for more information.

When People Just Don't Understand

Lack of support can make you sad, mad, or both. If people
don't understand, or can't be supportive, try to accept them for who
they are and what they can give. Sometimes lines need to be drawn.
It might be better to distance yourself from a relationship with someone who is actively critical of how your needs and abilities have
changed.

You may have to make some difficult judgment calls. Again, we
wish these situations didn't happen, but they do.

Control What You Can

There are books that tell you in global terms that life will be
better once you're in control, but this isn't one of them. Things happen that you can't control, both with and without Sjögren's syndrome. Sometimes it feels as if the disease is in control, and that isn't
a good feeling. Some researchers believe that one way to deal with
the lack of control is to develop an interest in an area where you do
have control (Hafen et al. 1996). You won't cure your illness, but
you *will* have something that helps restore your sense of competence
and worth.

A sense of competence and control begins in childhood.
Attitudes learned early in life influence how you deal with illness. It is

important to remember that as an adult, you have many more resources than you had as a child, and even if your first reaction is to be overwhelmed and panicked, you can subsequently regain more control. You can control the choices you make about treatment, the doctors you choose, the way you deal with family and friends, the ways in which you spend your time, and how you feel about yourself. You can learn to stay in control when things don't go well.

Optimism Helps

It helps to have a naturally optimistic temperament when living with a chronic disease. It's comforting to feel that everything will be all right in the end. As we have said, healthy people tend to overvalue themselves, while depressed people skew events negatively.

What if you are not an optimistic person? What if you are a dyed-in-the-wool pessimist? You can deliberately work at not always seeing the worst-case scenario. Stop yourself from thinking catastrophic thoughts, or if you think of them, put them aside. Ask yourself how an optimist might think. Alternatively, just accept that you are the way you are, but consider the alternative perspectives.

Make Time for Exercise

Exercise keeps muscles from atrophying, increases range of motion, and increases flexibility in both body and mind. For some, there is a spiritual side to exercise too; it is literally good for the soul. Some kinds of repetitive exercise can be like meditation.

Exercise doesn't have to be strenuous. It can be mild, gentle, and pleasurable. We don't subscribe to the "no pain, no gain" theory. Even mild exercise increases energy and well-being. It clears the mind and increases the sense of control.

Some people with Sjögren's have trouble with exercise, so the key is finding something that is right for you and not doing too much too soon, or even exercising under the supervision of a physical therapist. We suggest finding an activity you like, and if possible, doing it with someone. The presence of another person provides an impetus to get up and go on those days when you don't feel like it. You might try a dual exercise program, for days when you feel well and days when you don't.

Exercise is more than just physical activity. It relieves stress, anxiety, and depression. Even if it's moderate, exercise can feel like an accomplishment.

Make Time for Laughter

Once, a long time ago, a physician asked one of us, "What are you doing for fun?" The question seemed ludicrous. Who has time for fun when you're feeling exhausted, stressed, miserable, and, most of all, sick? What is there to laugh about? The physician's point was that if fun and laughter are missing from your life, their absence makes things much worse.

Laughter is healing and good for the soul. When you laugh, you shake off whatever is bothering you for that moment in time and space. When you stop laughing, the effects of the laughter linger, even if only for a while. Keep your sense of humor. It will be one of your best friends, even when no one else is around.

Touch and Passion

Touch, passionate and otherwise, is essential to humans. Touch is the earliest connection we have with those we love. When humans are deprived of touch, health can suffer. Children in institutions who were rarely touched in a loving way often suffered from failure to thrive. Even for those who live without a partner, there are ways to touch and be touched. You can get a massage, hug a child or a friend, or get a dog. Touch has been found to normalize irregular heartbeat, may lower blood pressure, and soothes anxiety and depression (Hafen et al. 1996). However, the therapeutic value of touch appears to depend on who is doing the touching and how it is interpreted. Ornstein and Sobel (1989) note that a comforting touch from a nurse can slow heart rate, but a touch associated with an anxiety-provoking procedure, such as an injection performed by the same nurse, can increase heart rate and produce an irregular heartbeat.

The touch of a sexual partner is more than just an expression of passion. It reassures, invigorates, and connects two people so that they become more than separate beings.

Not all love is passionate, and not all passion is directed at relationships with partners. Love between family members, friends, and parent and child is just as important and health-promoting as the love of a lover or spouse. The birth of a child or a grandchild fills you with love, hope, and a sense of affirmation and continuity. Pursuing activities you love gives you both satisfaction and sensory and emotional pleasure. People are passionate about all kinds of things, books, antiques, theater, travel, sports, art, and music among them. An activity like exercise or eating produces endorphins, neurochemicals that our brains produce in response to a variety of pleasurable circumstances. The production of endorphins increases our sense of pleasure, calm, and well-being and decreases feelings of stress and distress.

Maintain a Normal Life

As much as possible, try to maintain a normal life. We are not suggesting that life will be the same as it was before you were diagnosed or that you should ignore your illness. We are not suggesting you pretend that things are fine when they are not. It's not normal to have to give up a career, curtail activities that you love to pursue, take multiple medications, live with pain, and go to the doctor frequently. Most people don't have to spend long periods of time resting, or have to rest between each activity while still in their thirties, forties, or even fifties. They don't have frequent pain, infections that don't get better in a reasonable amount of time, or one medical problem after another. It's not normal to live with a disease that other people don't understand. You will continually wonder what might happen next, even if your condition is mild.

Living with Sjögren's syndrome will never be the same as living without it. Nevertheless, we suggest it's important to establish some way of living with it that includes the important elements of normal life—love and work. If you can't work, find something you like to do, something that you find meaningful, and do it when you can. If you can't make dinner for friends, invite friends over for a potluck or meet them in a restaurant. If you like to travel but can't take long trips, plan short ones. Be an armchair traveler; read books if you can't go anywhere at all. Cultivate activities you can do. There are lots of things to do in this world, and no one can do everything. The hard part is giving something up because of this disease. Don't let your feelings about that prevent you from finding other things that will make you feel that your life is larger than just your illness.

Remember that it takes time to develop a new "normal."

Maintain Your Self-Esteem

It's frustrating not to be able to do what you were able to do before you got sick. When your energy is limited, you don't feel like yourself, at least the self you used to know. It's reasonable to grieve for things once enjoyed that can no longer be continued, or that have to be given up because you can't do them now. Many people have trouble redefining themselves at retirement. Once they give up their professional life, they feel they are not who they were. It follows that people who are forced to give up activities before they are ready to also grieve for those losses.

This feeling of "I'm not who I was" can go along with chronic illness. On the other hand, as you age, you change.

Illness offers opportunity for authenticity even as it strips away activity. You are a person who is a mother, father, daughter, sister, brother, wife, husband, lover, or friend. Even if you don't do all the things as a mother that you did before you developed Sjögren's, ask your children, you will always be their mother!

Slowing down allows you to appreciate things that you might not have noticed when you were too busy to see them. You literally may have more time to listen to the birds and smell the flowers, and derive pleasure from them. You may have to give up some things, but you can gain others. While there are things that we had to give up because of having Sjögren's, there are other aspects of our lives that would not have happened without it—this book for example.

It's not always easy to be positive about the changes in identity and changes to your sense of self that go along with Sjögren's syndrome. It is important to keep a sense of the things that you can do, even when you are temporarily unable to do them. When you feel better, get back to them as soon as possible. Take advantage of small challenges. Too tired to walk a mile today? If you can do it tomorrow, you will feel a sense of accomplishment. Think about who you really are and what's important to you in life. It may be that you can't fly around the world, but you may help someone a little closer to home and, in the process, help yourself.

It is normal to compare yourself to others. You see what others have, and you want what they have. There will always be someone who has an easier life, a more expensive house, a better job, or someone who can do things you can't. There will also always be someone who has a more difficult life, whose limitations are more severe than your own. Try not to make comparisons. Compare yourself to yourself instead. If you are your own yardstick, you will have a better sense of where you are relative to where you were, and relative to where you want to be.

Keep Your Sense of Adventure

We also recommend not letting Sjögren's syndrome kill your sense of challenge and adventure. Life is much better when you are challenged. The nature of your challenges and adventures may change, but they are still out there. Things you would almost certainly have passed over before may intrigue you more now. For example, attending a conference on Sjögren's syndrome several years ago was an adventure for both of us. That's where we met, and we have each traveled extensively since then. Writing the book has been an adventure, too, of an unexpected and serendipitous kind.

People who love travel continue to love it, whether or not they have Sjögren's. Felicity Tompkins, of New Zealand, has had Sjögren's and rheumatoid arthritis for more than thirty years. Originally told by her doctor that she would have to quit taking trips, Felicity ignored his advice and developed her own system for traveling with Sjögren's. The fact that she lives in New Zealand means that many destinations in Europe and the United States require long hours of airplane travel. Felicity has the following suggestions. She carries:

* an extra cushion

* plenty of artificial tears

* a water bottle

* chewing gum (sugar free, of course)

* sunglasses to protect eyes from glare

* nasal spray

* a down pillow in her suitcase

* a folding director's chair

* an air mattress and a wool mattress cover

She carries these items in a large bag she had made for that purpose. She also carries a letter from her physician that explains she needs these extras and says she has never been charged for transporting these items.

We also recommend:

* carrying all your medications in either your purse or carry-on luggage

* taking an additional supply of medication to be packed in checked luggage

* carrying food and water, especially on plane trips

* making frequent stops if possible

* keeping a flexible itinerary when possible, so that you don't have to go if you don't feel up to it

* allowing extra time to recover from traveling

* talking with your doctor about what to do if you get sick while traveling

* carrying a MedicAlert bracelet, especially if you are traveling alone and to a country where you do not speak the language

* taking a list of your medications

For some people, having a chronic illness brings nothing but despair and depression. Others manage to keep on growing, even if their growth goes in an unexpected direction. It's important to do things that make you feel valued and that maintain your sense of who you are. Illness can force people to strip away the pretension and unnecessary things from their lives. It forces you to confront the fact that you are here for a limited time and that you may not get and do everything you want. Decide what is really important and go for it.

Be True to Yourself

Sick or well, it takes extra energy to be someone you're not. You don't have to be happy about the limitations that having Sjogren's necessitates, nor do you have to pretend everything is fine. Authenticity is a great gift. Give yourself permission to feel whatever it is that you are feeling. It's easier to get on with life once you and everyone else can openly acknowledge what is happening.

Some people feel that chronic illness provides an opportunity to reflect on what is really important in life. They see it as a chance to become more genuine and strip away the conventional but extraneous trappings of life. They travel, fall in love, pursue their interests, live well, and enjoy life, although they do not live the same life they would have lived without Sjögren's. Make sure to step out of the box and challenge yourself once in a while. It is still true that living well is the best revenge.

10

Healing

Healing can come from many sources. When we first started outlining this chapter, we thought about all the different kinds of therapy: individual and family therapy, intensive, supportive, and cognitive-behavioral psychotherapy, art therapy, music therapy, diet, nutrition, alternative and complementary therapies, yoga, acupuncture, physical therapy, and more that might be appropriate for people with Sjögren's syndrome. The list was so extensive, it appeared that the chapter would be nothing more than a brief and unsatisfactory paragraph about each.

Therapy is one way of healing, or trying to heal, but it isn't the only way. We decided to make this chapter primarily about the concept of healing, and about the ways to heal. Throughout this book, we have made the distinction between healing and being cured. Although there is not yet a cure for Sjögren's, the goal is to remain as healthy as possible and have peace of mind. You can find ways to get past problems and work towards peace of mind.

The concept of healing is a subjective one. What is healing to you may do nothing for someone else. The methods you choose depend to some extent on what is available to you and what resources you have, but many different healing modalities are widely accessible. Consider the broad spectrum and decide what you would be willing to do. Take a proactive approach. Things can and do get better if you work at them. Some people may use a single method, like meditation. Others prefer a variety: massage, exercise, diet, and creative activities.

We offer the following bit of advice: healing involves trying new things. Some will work, and some will not. You won't know what will work for you until you try something. For example, spending a day at the beach staring at the waves may be healing, unless of course, you are photosensitive and the sun makes you sick. A walk in the woods listening to the birds may help you connect with nature and remember that the world is a place of beauty. It may take you out of your own problems and make you feel better. You may not know, unless you have tried it, that meditation can help you when you are anxious. Unless you have attended a stress-reduction program or a support group, you may not know whether either would benefit you. If something doesn't work, don't give up. Try something else. When you approach the world with a fighting spirit and a sense that you can do something to make things better, you have started to heal.

There are many discussions of healing that make it sound like something that is possible to achieve in a perfect way. It probably isn't. There are always rough edges of reality that will never go away. Healing is a goal, as well as an imperfect state of being. No one is ever completely healed. You can feel better. The word heal is at the root of the word health. This might suggest that a healthy person is someone who is healed or who is someone who has never had anything from which they needed to heal. That would be wrong. We all gather wounds along the way, some big, others small.

The Power of Belief

The power of the placebo effect has been well documented in many studies. You believe that something will make you well, and your health improves as a result. Norman Cousins, the editor of the *Saturday Review,* wrote about how his health improved after large amounts of vitamin C and videos that made him laugh, despite the fact that he had been told that his condition was almost certainly degenerative (Cousins 1979). Cousins says that it is possible that his methods were only a placebo, but it doesn't matter. What matters is that he believed they would work for him, and he improved against the odds.

Just because symptoms respond to a placebo does not make them any less real. Placebos have been useful in relieving symptoms of "colds, headaches, seasickness, angina, anxiety, and post-operative pain" (Hafen et al. 1996, 433). The fact that this is so indicates the power of your beliefs and expectations and the importance of the connection between mind and body. It is important to remember that as the physiological connections between mind and body are better understood, the split between the two becomes increasingly artificial and obsolete.

Belief can also work against you. This is called the *nocebo* effect (Benson 1996). If the placebo effect speaks to the power of positive expectations, the nocebo effect describes how negative expectations may become self-fulfilling prophecies. In *The Lost Art of Healing,* Dr. Bernard Lown (1996) tells the story of a woman who was told by another doctor that she had a condition called "TS." These initials stood for a heart condition known as tricuspid stenosis, but the patient assumed that "TS" meant "terminal situation" and understood the doctor's words to mean that she was going to die. Although Dr. Lown later tried to clarify the diagnosis and reassure the patient, he could not convince her.

Within a very short time, to Dr. Lown's horror, the woman's lungs filled with fluid and she died. Her death was not representative of her diagnosis of tricuspid stenosis; something else had killed her. Dr. Lown attributed the patient's death to her belief that her situation was terminal. He could do nothing to save her.

Authenticity As Healing

One of the things about living with an invisible illness is that there is always a dilemma about how to present yourself. There is often a split between the way you present yourself and the way you feel inside. You say you are fine when you feel sick with worry, or just plain sick. You smile when you want to cry. You conform to the expectations of other people and the norms of your culture. Sometimes you do this to an extreme. You say you are fine when you are running a high fever. You go to an important meeting when it is more important for you to be home in bed, or you attend a dinner party when you are too nauseous to eat. You tell no one you are sick; you don't want to be judged as incompetent or weak. You don't know when to quit. As one woman with Sjögren's said, "I walk around with things that would send other people to the emergency room."

Living in a way that is not authentic eventually takes a toll. One woman (who asked not to be identified), said that one of the best things about going on disability was that it allowed her to reclaim her life. If she did not feel well, she could say so. If she could not do something that day, she could postpone it until she felt well enough to get it done. "Authenticity," she said, "was an unbelievable luxury after so many years of smiling and saying I was fine when I felt horrid. It was a relief to be able to admit it even to myself. I could stop when I needed to. Being genuine with myself enabled me to be more so with others, and I found that they were, for the most part, more understanding than I thought."

She noted that this feeling of authenticity came only after she had announced to the world that she had an illness that was serious enough to disrupt her life. She had kept it hidden or minimized it for many years. When she left a high-level job on disability, many of her colleagues had no idea that there was anything medically wrong. Those who did know assumed that she had some medical problems that were only intermittently significant. The reality was that she had pushed herself beyond her limits for years. "Once I left my job," she said, "I was able to accept who I am now. I did not have to pretend to be someone I had been, but no longer was. I didn't have to pretend to have energy that I didn't have. I could stop and rest when I needed to. I'm only sorry that the combination of the way I felt and the way the system worked did not allow me to do it sooner, before I got so sick that it became impossible for me to do anything at all."

Letting Go

Letting go of old expectations is another step on the path to healing. The woman above, who was pleased that giving up her job allowed her to be more authentic and more herself, was unhappy about the fact that she would never know the full extent of where her career might have taken her. She was eventually able to accept this fact, although initially it caused her a great deal of distress. The increased wholeness that she felt after leaving her job did not mitigate her grief, but in time, she accepted her loss as the trade she had to make. She let go of the career she had in order to take better care of herself. This allowed her to pursue other avenues in her life. In the process, she was able to better accept herself and her Sjögren's.

Being able to let go is an accomplishment. It is useful not to hold on to anger or past expectations. Instead, focus on present accomplishments. Anger and disappointment are by no means necessarily illness-related; they are experiences known to everyone. Not holding on to bad experiences is also useful when you deal with lack of caring and compassion in the medical establishment. When something you wanted doesn't work out, it helps to be able to let it go and just move on.

Releasing expectations and letting go is not always something you do solo. It is often interactive and interpersonal. Other people's expectations are based on what they perceive you to be capable of doing. Their perceptions are also influenced by what they need from you. If you never modify the image you project, never publicly try to accommodate the disease in any way, neither will anyone else.

Even if you make it clear that things have changed, others may be slow to follow. But they will most certainly not understand and adapt unless you lead the way. It might be hard to show weakness, but the cost of always being competent is that others will expect it. They will not realize that there are times when you cannot fulfill all your obligations.

For many people with Sjögren's, there is always some medical problem to deal with, and both the symptoms and the process of dealing with these problems are exhausting, frustrating, and traumatic. A chronic disease can bring nonstop stress. It is important to find ways to release it whenever possible. The goal is to maximize the stress-free intervals, and to deal with the stressful ones as expediently as possible. Sometimes, and here we are referring to any kind of ongoing stress, it feels as if healing takes places in the cracks, those stress-free intervals between one crisis and another.

Cognitive Restructuring

Letting go involves cognitive restructuring. You have to learn to think about something differently, or see it from a different perspective. Since stress is based largely on perception, it involves becoming aware of what you are thinking and feeling.

Thoughts and feelings can be obvious, subliminal, or even unconscious. Often thoughts and feelings we are not aware of contribute strongly to the way we see and interact with the world. For example, when faced with an unpleasant procedure, if you are sure it will be frightening and painful, you are likely to experience it as such. Your expectations become a self-fulfilling prophecy.

In this case, you need to address your concerns so that they do not become reality. You can also differentiate between thoughts and fact, sometimes by doing something as simple as asking yourself whether something is a fear or whether it is real.

In *Full Catastrophe Living,* Jon Kabat-Zinn (1990) suggests different ways to attend to your internal life more fully. His methods enable you to become aware of the full extent of what you are thinking and feeling. He emphasizes both observation and detachment. "I am feeling anxious," is not necessarily the same as "I am anxious," he says. If you are feeling anxious, you can take a problem-focused approach and attend to the reason for the anxiety. At times when a problem-focused approach doesn't work (for example, when you talk with the doctor about a procedure but are anxious anyway), he recommends staying with the feelings and acknowledging them for what they are.

Another suggestion is to differentiate between the thoughts surrounding something and the phenomenon itself. The example that Kabat-Zinn gives is pain. A person may have all sorts of thoughts (and fears) about pain, he says, but these are not the same as the pain itself. This is a useful differentiation in regard to living with Sjögren's syndrome. You may have all sorts of thoughts and feelings about having Sjögren's: "I hate this disease." "It is ruining my life." "I can't stand it." "I hate having to deal with all these medications and doctors." "I'll never do the things I want to do." These are only a few examples of upsetting thoughts about Sjögren's, but these thoughts about the disease are not the same as the disease itself.

Domar and Dreher (1996) suggest that you ask yourself why you assumed a particular idea, whether it is accurate, and whether thinking in this way contributes to the amount of stress that you are feeling. Once you begin to monitor your thoughts, they say, you may realize that certain recognizable patterns emerge. For example, you may recognize that the anxiety you feel is often worse than the actuality of a given situation. When you become aware of your patterns of thinking, you can begin to question whether these thoughts and ways of thinking contribute to or detract from your general sense of well-being. This doesn't mean you have to take a Pollyanna attitude. According to Domar and Dreher (1996), cognitive restructuring is not meant to hide painful truths but to address what keeps you from dealing with reality in a more complete and effective way, without being restricted by unnecessary negativity.

Chronic Stress Takes a Toll

As we have said, stress is an inevitable fact of life. No one is exempt; no one can avoid it. Stress may come from both good and bad things, but, according to Dr. Esther Sternberg, a rheumatologist at the National Institutes of Health, there is a difference between stress that is short-lived and stress that is chronic. Sternberg (2001) points out that chronic stress is more likely to impair the immune system because your body has no chance to recover from the physiologic changes of the stress response. Especially for people with autoimmune diseases, relentless stress can be a burden on an already impaired immune system.

When stress is not continuous, even if it is severe, your body has a chance to recover. Unfortunately, with an autoimmune disease such as Sjögren's, a physical health crisis can precipitate other emotional and life crises, and the immune system has no chance to recover. Perhaps this is why people with Sjögren's syndrome and other autoimmune diseases often experience flares when they have to deal with unremitting stress. Many people have noted that flares occur just after a prolonged stressful situation.

In *Full Catastrophe Living,* Kabat-Zinn (1990) describes a state of hyperarousal that is both physiological and psychological in nature. He notes that this can become a permanent state, accompanied by increased muscle tension, blood pressure, headaches, exhaustion, sleep disorders, and psychological distress. As therapists who work with post-traumatic stress patients know, it is often difficult for such people to differentiate between minor and major stresses. They respond to both in the same way.

Mindfulness and the Relaxation Response

Increased and continuous stress leads to a state of hyperarousal. To offset this, it is important to develop mechanisms to quiet the body and mind. Kabat-Zinn (1990) outlines a method for taking control by using a technique he calls "mindfulness." Cardiologist Herb Benson (1996) and psychologist Alice Domar (Domar and

Dreher 1996) both suggest using the "relaxation response." The idea behind each technique is to slow down the body and mind, to live fully in the present, and provide an opportunity for increased well-being and healing.

Both mindfulness and the relaxation response have been widely used with people who have many different physical problems: migraines, backaches, cardiac problems, cancer, and infertility. They have helped people recover from disabling accidents and cope with serious illness, and they should be helpful to people with Sjögren's and other autoimmune diseases as well.

Hospitals in many parts of the country have mind-body programs that teach mindfulness, the relaxation response, and other forms of stress reduction. Benson originated the relaxation response, a technique that is elegant in its simplicity and usefulness. According to Benson (1996), there are only two steps to follow. The first is to repeat a word or prayer that has some meaning to you. While breathing slowly, repeat the word you have chosen. If intrusive thoughts interrupt you (as they are likely to do), disregard them and continue breathing. Ideally, you should be in a comfortable, quiet place, and this technique should be practiced from ten to twenty minutes once or twice a day.

The result is a quieting of the mind and body, and a chance to counteract the effects of stress and hyperarousal. This technique is also helpful as a way of preparing for medical procedures or surgery, or as a way of dealing with the stress and anxiety of waiting for test results. Mindfulness, meditation, and the relaxation response are all ways of being fully present in the moment, and they allow access to subliminal thoughts and feelings.

Although these techniques sound simple, they are not. They require practice. As anyone who has ever used the Lamaze technique in preparation for childbirth knows, the desired response doesn't just happen. It takes work to elicit the relaxation response. Look for a mind-body program in your area if you are interested in learning about these techniques. If one is not available, you can find a variety of books and tapes that are useful guides.

When so much feels out of control, programs like these give you a way of taking back some control and give you an enhanced sense of well-being. As anyone who has had this kind of experience knows, achieving calm where panic once was leads to a new perspective. Mindfulness is a way of being who you are where you are, whatever state you find yourself in. It is a way of living fully in the moment. If you are able to do this, you are bound to feel an increased sense of acceptance about your life.

Living with a chronic illness becomes easier once you accept the illness as part of your life, but that doesn't mean it is easy. Sometimes the struggle is in the foreground, sometimes it recedes, but for some, it is always a struggle. It is healing to take control.

Slowing Down

Living in the slow lane can be the most difficult thing some of us ever have to do. It is an ongoing source of frustration to have to live at a slower pace. Slowing down and accepting a new pace is difficult. While some people are relieved, others continue to miss a faster-paced life. However, when you learn to live at your own pace, you learn something about being authentic. Slowing down is a goal for most people. For those with Sjögren's, it can be a necessity.

Faith and Prayer

Those who believe in God have always relied on faith to sustain them through difficult times. Comfort and healing are fundamental to all religions. You may have a favorite prayer that you use when you feel the need, or you may have attended a healing service at your church or synagogue. Words with religious significance may also be used to elicit the relaxation response (Benson 1996). Such words can be recited while walking, for what is called a "walking meditation." They can also be used during some other repetitive activity, such as swimming. One of us uses them whenever having blood drawn. It relieves the tension and anxiety and actually reduces the sense of pain.

Religion can make you part of a community and give you a sense of purpose and belonging. Talking with a rabbi or priest comforted people with illness long before therapy was invented. Even those who have never considered themselves religious sometimes find that a connection to their spirituality can become more important when they are diagnosed with a significant health problem.

One recent interesting phenomenon described by Benson (1996) is intercessory prayer. Benson describes a study in which one group of patients in a coronary care unit of a hospital had someone praying for them while another group did not. The patients were unaware anyone was praying on their behalf; however, at the end of the study, those patients who had been prayed for suffered fewer complications and required less medication. No explanation is offered, but it's interesting to contemplate that perhaps the healing power of prayer was at least partially responsible.

Psychotherapy and Healing

Psychotherapy helps healing by providing ways to cope with illness, come to terms with it, find ways to live with it, and examine identity in the face of it. It also helps provide new ways to deal with anxiety, uncertainty, depression, loss, and changes in relationships that occur as a result of living with Sjögren's syndrome. Psychotherapy can be short-term, long-term, ongoing, or intermittent. It can be supportive, interpretive, cognitive-behavioral, individual, group, or family in orientation.

The kind of mental health care that many people have access to depends on their health insurance, and all too often, this is a relatively short-term benefit. However, even if you have only six or seven sessions covered by your insurance company, you can derive some benefit from short-term treatment.

It is important to find a therapist familiar with chronic illness. He or she should understand something about the physical nature of Sjögren's and be able to appreciate the impact of it on your life. Since healing in psychotherapy will probably be based on finding an attentive and empathic presence in another person, find someone with whom you feel comfortable and can speak freely. This person doesn't have to be an expert on Sjögren's syndrome, but it is not unreasonable to expect your therapist to learn something about it.

Individual Therapies

Almost any kind of therapy can be valuable, so how is a person to choose? In part, it depends on what you think you need. If you want a relationship with a therapist that will last, find a mental health professional who will work with you over the long term, even if you only need to see this person intermittently. If you think you will need medication for anxiety or depression, you can either be treated by a psychiatrist or be referred to one by a psychologist, social worker, or licensed mental health worker.

Short-term therapy helps deal with focal or limited issues and may be for only a few weeks. Therapy may be repeated whenever there is a need.

Supportive psychotherapy helps you deal with ongoing stressful issues and fosters your own coping skills. It may also help you develop new ones. Supportive psychotherapy generally takes place on a weekly basis, but may be either more or less frequent, as circumstances require. It generally deals with events in the present, but may also integrate the past with the present.

Exploratory or integrative psychotherapy usually places more emphasis on integrating past experiences into the present and helps place present reactions in the context of your life experiences. It may take place more than once a week and has also been called intensive psychotherapy. It is not psychoanalysis, but it has some similarities in terms of the intense nature of the relationship between patient and therapist.

Cognitive-behavioral therapy may be used to deal with a specific problem, such as panic attacks, or may be used more generally, as in the treatment of depression. It places emphasis on thoughts, perceptions, and their relationship to both emotion and behavior. Cognitive therapy can have a narrow focus—it can address a specific issue—or it can be used in a broader context, such as looking at negative thoughts and feelings that make it difficult to deal with a particular set of experiences. Some cognitive-behavioral therapists use desensitization to help you become less anxious. Therapists may also use other tools, such as hypnosis. Make sure the therapist you choose is appropriately trained. It's perfectly acceptable to ask questions about a therapist's training and experience in any area. A therapist should answer such questions candidly and without reservation.

Family Therapy

While individual psychotherapy is an excellent way for you to focus on your own thoughts and feelings about Sjögren's syndrome, family therapy may also be helpful. In this situation, a therapist facilitates discussion of issues that might otherwise be difficult and troublesome.

Many family therapists will begin with the whole family and see individual members during the course of the relationship. A good family therapist moderates and paces the context of sessions in order to minimize the feeling that "if we talk about this, it will get out of control."

Group Therapy

Group therapy provides an excellent way to see how other people deal and cope with illness and other life events. In a group, you are exposed to a variety of people whose situations vary. Support groups vary widely in focus. Some meet on a regular basis for ongoing support, while others meet only a few times a year. Some have a structure, such as a speaker; others are free-form discussions. Therapy groups always meet on a regular basis and are usually less structured. They focus on the interaction of the group members as well as the content of group discussion. If the nature of a group doesn't feel appropriate to you, see if another one is available. The nature of a group often depends very much on the style and philosophy of its leader.

Alternative and Complementary Therapies

Alternative and *complementary* are terms that are sometimes used interchangeably in describing therapies, but they really have different meanings. Whereas alternative therapy is used in place of conventional therapy, complementary therapy is used as an adjunct to conventional therapy. For example, acupuncture may be considered an alternative therapy when it is used in lieu of pain medication. When used in addition to one of the nonsteroidal anti-inflammatory medications or some other pain medication, it becomes a complementary therapy. Some forms of alternative therapies have little evidence to back them up, while others, such as acupuncture, have been used in other countries for thousands of years. The relaxation response and the use of mindfulness described above are both complementary therapies.

The rise of interest in both alternative and complementary therapies may be the result of the increasingly impersonal nature of medical practice. A physical therapist, a massage therapist, or a psychologist who teaches the relaxation response knows you over time and may know as much about you as your physician but has a different perspective. They may not know about the numbers on lab tests, but they know about how an individual's body feels when it is hurting and what changes when things improve. They also take more time to talk. The combination of therapy and the development of a close relationship is healing. The Arthritis Foundation has published a *Guide to Alternative Therapies* (Horstman 1999). Some of the topics addressed in this book are the healing power of touch, diet, herbal remedies, exercise, the mind-body connection, and the role of prayer and spirituality in healing.

Express Yourself

Expressive therapies using art, music, dance, or writing can also help you heal. Rita Nathanson, an art therapist and potter who lives in Illinois, talks about her work with patients who have both physical and emotional illnesses:

> We're all pretty good at expressing ourselves verbally but our images can also be a powerful way to express and explore feelings, helping us to identify and understand ourselves on deeper levels, as well as to communicate what we are feeling. Art is a here-and-now experience, accessible to everyone, regardless of talent or expertise. Because we are the expert on how we feel, making art in the service of self expression and exploration can never be "wrong." Drawing, painting, collage, or using clay to explore images as metaphor and symbol is both a means to express feelings and to look at them more objectively. It communicates what we are about to friends, families, and even our doctors, as well as to ourselves. We become both the maker and the observer of personal imagery. (2002)

Recently someone asked one of us whether writing this book had been healing. "Yes," was the immediate response. For both of us, it has been therapeutic to pull together so many of the thoughts and feelings of other people about their lives. Many have Sjögren's, but not all. It has been therapeutic to reread so much of the fine literature about illness that has been quoted in these pages.

We enjoyed getting to know some very brave people as they rise to life's challenges. Writing this book has enabled us to discover more about their thoughts and feelings as they shared how they live with Sjögren's from day to day, year to year. It has also given us a chance to examine our own thoughts and feelings about having Sjögren's. In some ways, we feel like "old hands," survivors, at least so far. We also know the uncertainty, challenge, and difficulty of struggling with it on a daily basis. We continue to wish it would go away, and know that it won't. We hope we have imparted information, perspective, and hope.

When you have Sjögren's you join a group of people who may have nothing in common but their disease. You join a club that will willingly accept you as a member, but it is a club you never imagined you would join. Since it isn't possible to resign your membership, you might as well learn all you can about what you are living with. You may find fellowship and comfort in knowing that there are others who will welcome you and extend a hand. You don't have to go it alone.

11

Work and Disability

What you do is a big part of who you are. You may work at a job
you love or hate, a job that lasts a few years or months, or the better
part of a lifetime. Most people, at some point, work outside the
home. One of the greatest social changes of the past three decades is
the increased entry of women into the workforce. Families with two
working parents have become the norm. Work is not necessarily
reimbursed. Although women are not paid for the work they do at
home, taking care of a family also constitutes work.

Work provides you with more than your identity. Unless you
are independently wealthy, the amount of money you earn defines
your lifestyle, the kind of house you have, the car you drive, where
your children go to school, where and what you eat, what kind of
recreation you enjoy and where you go when you travel. If a family
with two wage-earning parents suddenly becomes a single-income
family, the family's lifestyle changes. Depending on the size of the
second income, it may be an event of moderate or catastrophic
importance.

Not only does the amount of income change when you cut down or are forced to leave work, but your sense of self changes as well. Some important questions you may have are:

* "What will I do if I am unable to work?"

* "How will I take care of my family?"

* "Will I (we) be able to survive?"

* "Will I lead a meaningful life?"

* "How will I spend my time?"

The need to change or modify what you do depends on the extent of your disease and the nature of your work. Some people make few changes while others are forced to go on disability. Many people with Sjögren's continue to work full time. Many continue to do so even though it pushes them to their limit, and they must sacrifice other things in order to keep their jobs.

Some people have jobs or careers that allow them flexible hours or to work from home, but most work does not permit such flexibility. It would be difficult to be a surgeon who did not feel well enough to do an operation on the day and time it was scheduled, a nurse who could not take care of her patients, or a musician who could not show up for an evening performance.

Occupations are task driven. They depend on the ability of a worker to accomplish goals or get jobs done within a given period of time. This is true whether you work in a factory or an office or you are a physician in a hospital. If you cannot perform the duties of your job or occupation, you will meet some definitions of disability. If you cannot perform the duties of any job or occupation, you are likely to be considered disabled by even the most stringent criteria.

To Tell or Not to Tell?

You may wonder whether to disclose the fact that you have Sjögren's syndrome. You may wonder whether it will affect your chances of being hired, how it will affect your relationships with supervisors and coworkers, and whether it will affect your career track. Some people, afraid of negative consequences, say nothing. As long as their illness remains invisible, they do not choose to reveal its presence.

Although Sjögren's syndrome is largely invisible, it may not be easy to keep secret. Eyedrops, frequent trips to the bathroom, fatigue, diminished concentration, doctor's appointments, vulnerability to infection, delayed healing, and sudden changes in energy level are all open to scrutiny by coworkers or supervisors, especially if you require permission to leave for frequent doctor's appointments. Friends and coworkers may notice that you are inconsistent about carrying out job responsibilities and wonder why. They get over a cold or flu in a few days, while it takes you weeks. Coworkers and supervisors sometimes incorrectly attribute fluctuations in physical health to other causes, such as preoccupation with nonwork-related matters, marital problems, or depression.

The dilemma begins before you are hired. If you talk about your disease, will you ruin your chances of getting the job? If you believe that your disease will not impinge on your ability to do the job, there is not much of a problem. If you have been only recently diagnosed, you have no way of knowing how much of a problem Sjögren's will be.

The next point of choice is at the preemployment physical, if there is one. Although not always a prerequisite, many firms require physicals. Here you are asked about medical conditions, you wonder what will happen to any information that you give, and you also may wonder what will happen if you fail to disclose a preexisting condition. According to one labor lawyer we spoke with, the most important information for employers is whether or not you have a medical condition that will prevent you from doing your job. One very real dilemma is that Sjögren's may present no problems that would interfere with work over long periods of time. On the other hand, the stress of a new job may increase your vulnerability to medical problems. Whether or not you are more vulnerable than anyone else is a question only you can answer.

There are psychological aspects of the disclosure dilemma as well as legal and ethical ones. If you do not disclose your Sjögren's, you have to pretend to be fine when you are not, and appear energetic and interested when you feel just the opposite. Anyone may have a significant split between the way they feel inside and the face they show the world. Sjögren's has the potential to enlarge that gap between your public and private self. It can be difficult to sustain this split between the way you feel and the way you present yourself, especially if it is necessary to perpetuate this dichotomy for months or years.

We have no answer to the question of whether to tell or not to tell. We offer no advice. However, it is important to remember that under the terms of the Americans with Disabilities Act (ADA), you may not ask an employer to make any kind of modifications without disclosing what kind of physical (or emotional) problems you are having.

How Many Tasks Can You Handle?

Sjögren's often affects people at a time in their lives when they have multiple responsibilities. In addition to working, you may be a parent, a spouse, a caretaker for elderly parents, or all of the above. You wonder how you can deal with all of these different responsibilities and what the effect on your health will be. Multitasking is difficult for a normal person; it is even harder when you have a disease that worsens when you are under stress. It is easy to feel burdened, easy to become overwhelmed, upset, angry, or depressed.

There are times when it feels impossible to do everything. It is important to remember that if you get really sick, you won't be able to do much of anything. It's also important not to put yourself last, something many women do. Prioritize. You may be able to do one activity with your children but no more than that. You may be able to shop, but not cook. You may be able to do something on Saturday night, but only if you rest all afternoon (or all day). It may be necessary to reassign tasks within the family so that everyone helps out more.

What modifications can you make? We know people who have taken jobs that are closer to home or enable them to work from home, who have switched careers, who have chosen to work part-time, or who, when all else fails, have gone on disability in order to maintain and preserve their health. We also know, and here each of us can speak from personal experience, that sometimes the demands of work are accomplished at the expense of personal well-being.

There is a benefit to multitasking, wearing multiple hats, and having multiple identities. If you need to leave one, other aspects of your life remain intact. Perhaps this is why women have traditionally done better at retirement than men. Working women with families have always had multiple responsibilities. They have always been pulled in different (and often conflicting) directions.

Work and Money

What happens if you can't work? If you have disability insurance, it may pay a significant portion of the salary that you earned during the last calendar year that you worked. If you have a working spouse, you may be able to cut back on expenses and live on one salary or work part-time.

Carol had practiced for only five years when Sjögren's syndrome and lupus made it impossible for her to continue her work as a school psychologist. She is single and had enjoyed living on her own, but she could no longer afford it after she stopped working. When Carol returned to her parents' house, she found the adjustment painful and difficult. Although she comes from a close family, it was hard for her not to have her own space, and not to be able to come and go without having to check in with her parents. In some ways, it made her feel like a child again. Carol receives Social Security benefits, but not enough money to live on her own. She knows that she is fortunate to have a good and comfortable home, but it has been stressful for her to give up both the independence and the professional life she used to have.

Frieda was both more and less fortunate. Employed by a state agency that paid approximately two-thirds of her salary when she went on disability, she has been able to modify her lifestyle and continue to live a simple life. Unlike Carol, Frieda has no close family with whom she could live if it became necessary. She inherited a house from her parents and was able to rent out the small apartment that she owned to supplement her disability income. She has kept her independence, but since she no longer works, she finds that she spends a great deal of time alone. She is only forty-five, and all of her friends work.

When Kayla and her husband decided that it was no longer possible for him to work full time, they sold their home in the northeast and moved to Florida, where they were able to purchase a larger home for less money. Although reluctant to move far from friends and family, they have found that his health has improved in the warmer climate and they are enjoying a more relaxed lifestyle. They have made new friends and were surprised to find that they like their new life.

Age and stage of life make a difference in thinking about finances and financial planning. Here are some questions to ask yourself if you are considering leaving your job:

* Do you have a pension plan?

* Do you have investments?

* Do you have life insurance?

* Do you have a mortgage? Can you refinance? Or is your home free and clear?

* If you have no mortgage, can you afford your taxes?

* Is taking a reverse mortgage something you might consider?

* Could you live in a smaller home or apartment? Can you draw income from your home, perhaps by renting out a room or creating a small apartment for rent?

* What other assets do you have? Can they generate more income than they do now while maintaining a high level of safety?

* Is there some work you can do to add extra money if necessary?

* Are you willing to work at something completely different?

* Is there something that you have always wanted to do?

* Can you afford to volunteer?

* If you have worked as a volunteer in the past, is there some experience that might translate into a job?

It is worth sitting down with a financial planner and considering all your options. Financial planning is not a luxury; it is a necessity. Consider the worst-case scenario: "What would I (we) do if I couldn't work?"

If you are considering cutting down on the number of hours you work, keep in mind that if you have private or employment-related disability insurance, the amount you receive may be based on your last year's income. Some disability policies allow you to continue to earn up to a certain percent of your full-time salary. This is called a residual disability benefit, and not every disability policy has this provision. Check with your agent or the benefits person in your human resources department to find out what kind of coverage you have, and plan accordingly.

Work and Self-Esteem

Work done well generates a sense of effectiveness, which increases a person's sense of self-worth and self-esteem. If health-related problems interfere with accomplishments, the result may be a profound sense of loss, disappointment, or even shame. Because the drive to fulfill personal ambitions can be so strong, many people go to great lengths to carry on, despite feeling very sick. Sue was an academic who entered her field when she was thirty-three. At thirty-eight she acquired a tenure-track position at a college and was on her way to becoming known in her field. She had also just had a baby. When her daughter was three, she separated from her husband and was diagnosed with Sjögren's syndrome and possible lupus. Sue recounts her struggle to continue with both family and work life despite her disease:

> At first I made a few lifestyle changes, but not many.
> I worked hard and played hard. I was still doing very
> well. I managed to get enough publications to apply for
> tenure. . . . However, I was already beginning to feel some
> of the fatigue of Sjögren's. I was sapped of energy. I slept
> every spare moment at home. I was no longer bringing
> work home because I had no energy to do anything. I was
> barely able to do the necessary housework to keep things
> going. I consulted with my rheumatologist, who put me on
> Plaquenil and prednisone. I was never to be free from
> prednisone again. She encouraged me to grab naps at
> work if I could.
>   I ate lunch at my desk while working, then slept
> during the lunch hour. Unfortunately, I slept so deeply that
> I had to be shaken awake, so my naps were no secret.
> I was also missing work fairly often when I was simply too
> exhausted. I was agonizing about going to work when I was
> so exhausted, knowing I wouldn't have anything left for my
> daughter at the end of the day. . . . My ex-husband and I
> shared custody, so my daughter wasn't there every night.

I negotiated a partial disability leave so that I could work half-time. I was only able to work in this context for one year before I would have to return to work full time or go to part-time employment. I was obviously kissing tenure good-bye. This was a bitter pill. I was heartbroken and angry. I had just been asked to write a chapter for a highly regarded textbook. My work and interests were beginning to be noticed in the national community. But at work, I was fighting for my job and still missing work. I missed at least one day out of every two weeks, even though I was only assigned half-time.

Sue eventually decided that she needed to quit her job and apply for disability. Although she has been able to survive financially, there has been a lingering sense of disappointment and loss.

The decision to leave the college was very difficult. I struggled with feelings of shame, shame that I was going to allow someone else to support me. I had to share my decision with various colleagues and observe their reactions. To a one, they were sympathetic and seemed to acknowledge that I had no choice. This helped me to recognize that it was not a shameful thing but a matter of survival.

I was deeply disappointed at walking away from my plans and hopes. I went through most of this grieving before actually making the choice to leave. When I left, I still felt some loss. Mixed with that feeling, however, were feelings of relief that the ordeal was over. I had been pushing myself so hard for so long that I had not realized how punishing it was until I stopped.

An article by Jill Jordan Sieder (2000) notes that about 40 percent of people suffer some symptoms of depression at the time they leave work. As Sue demonstrated so clearly, the decision to go on disability is difficult and painful emotionally. The very word *disability* is distasteful, because it implies uselessness. It can feel as if you have failed, while it is really your body that has failed to keep up with the demands of the job, an important distinction. It helps to remember that although you may be unable to do your job, you are still a person with a variety of abilities, talents, gifts, and aptitudes. If you are forced to go on disability or to retire sooner than you would like because of illness, keep that in mind.

Enforced or Early Retirement

In addition to providing a salary, the ability to work makes you feel normal. "As long as I can work, I know I can't be that sick," one woman said, even as she acknowledged that she was losing ground, and didn't know how much longer she would be able to keep up the pace of her very pressured job.

Most people plan for retirement, but not many plan to retire because they are unable to work. While healthy friends joke about wishing they did not have to work, or remark about how difficult it is to have to juggle work and other responsibilities, they do not realize what a black hole leaving a job or profession prematurely can be. If you can't work because you are sick and someone tells you how envious they are, they don't understand the whole picture. All they see is that you don't have to get up and go to work. They are oblivious to the fact that you *can't* work.

For a healthy person, it's hard to understand that working just isn't possible. They don't understand what it is like to find it difficult to summon the energy to brush your teeth or get dressed, to be too tired to eat, talk, or concentrate. They wouldn't like it if they had to spend every afternoon resting, or if they got sick and didn't get better. People who have never had any health problems may wonder if you are faking it or if you are depressed. They may think you are just not trying hard enough.

It can be troublesome to be "retired" when everyone else gets up and goes to work in the morning. It leaves a void where a purpose once was. It can break your heart to leave a job that you love because you are unable to do it. Healthy friends or relatives who have the fantasy of a permanent vacation have just that—a fantasy. When people make remarks like, "You're so lucky you don't have to work," or "Don't you think you could work if you really wanted to?" it is safe to assume they are really not talking about the reality of living with Sjögren's syndrome.

If you are forced to leave work or retire early, try the following:

* Give yourself time to recover your energy. Most people are exhausted by the time they decide to leave work. Allow enough time to find your baseline. Once you have it, you will know what you are able to do.

* Allow yourself to grieve. The situation warrants it. You may return to work at some time in the future, or you may not.

Either way, you have had to do something that you didn't wish to do. Some people grieve before they leave work, while they are making the decision. For others, the feelings and the process of grieving is something that continues for a long time.

* Recognize that you need to reconstruct your life, but this can be done over time, not all at once. Some people feel a tremendous void; others do not.

* Look for other ways to occupy your time, but don't rush into activity. Think about how you feel and what you feel able to do. Clip articles from the newspaper or magazines about things that interest you or that describe how others have negotiated this transition. Look for things that will have some meaning for you. You may want to start with something simple—like taking a walk with a friend every morning.

* Volunteer if you can. Many new careers have grown out of activities that were initially performed for only a few hours a week. Volunteering not only helps you feel good about yourself, but it introduces you to new people and skills.

* Keep up contacts with family and friends. Make new friends. This means that you will have to participate in some activity where you meet people. Don't isolate yourself. Relationships are very important during any transition.

* Try not to see leaving work as just an ending. Remember that when doors close, windows open.

Of course, not everyone grieves over leaving their work. You may say to yourself: "I did my job for twenty years, and I couldn't wait to get out of there. I feel so much better now that I'm not working. My health is better and I can do what I want. What's done is done." If this is you, we are glad that the process has been simple and straightforward. Consider yourself fortunate that the transition was so smooth.

Disability Benefits

Disability insurance is either offered through your employer or is something you have purchased on your own, through an individual agent or insurance company. If you have a group policy, a pre-existing condition may not matter, or you may be excluded because of it. If you have coverage through your workplace, your employer generally pays part or all of the premium. The benefits from these policies are usually taxed.

In certain cases, it may be possible to have both individual and group benefits. Perhaps you purchased an individual policy before you went to work at a company or institution. While working there, you decided to continue paying your individual policy although you were also allowed disability benefits through the company plan. Check with both your agent and human resources representative to make sure that in the event you are forced to go on disability, you can receive benefits from both policies. It is also advisable to ask about any preexisting condition clause your policy might contain. You need to know whether your policy includes a residual disability clause that allows you to do some work and earn some percentage of your former salary while on disability, and you need to understand how your insurance company defines "disability." Does it mean not being able to perform the duties of your own profession or occupation, or must you be unable to perform any sort of work at all?

Social Security

The Social Security Administration (SSA) has two programs that provide disability benefits. Social Security Disability Insurance (SSDI) pays benefits to those who have worked enough and paid enough Social Security taxes to meet the criteria. Supplemental Security Income (SSI) pays benefits based on financial need. When you apply for either program, the SSA collects medical and other information about you in order to make a determination about benefits. The SSA Web site offers an extensive array of information about the process of applying, and how the decisions are made.

The SSA uses the strict definition of disability. Defined this way, disability is the inability to perform any substantial gainful activity as a result of physical or emotional impairment. There is also an expectation that the impairment will last for a continuous period of at least twelve months. The "impairment" must be determined and corroborated by objective medical evidence such as signs and symptoms that your physician has observed and treated, and laboratory abnormalities that have shown up repeatedly in blood tests, X rays, MRI scans, and so on.

According to Sieder (2000), a variety of steps are possible if your initial claim is denied by the SSA. Applications for disability are frequently denied on the first try and subsequently approved. You can request a reconsideration, and if it is denied, you can proceed to request a hearing before an administrative law judge. She also notes that it is helpful if you have been diagnosed with one or more conditions that have been listed in the official list of medical impairments, which is available from the SSA or available from the SSA's Web site.

The SSA has the right to review your claim periodically to make sure that your health has not changed. Once on disability, you do have the right to earn some money while receiving Social Security benefits, and there is a trial period that allows you to go back to work without losing benefits.

If you are denied benefits, you may file the initial appeal on your own, or you may want to hire an attorney. Sieder (2000) suggests hiring an attorney with an expertise in disability law. Many attorneys will work on a contingency basis so that their fee is deducted from your initial award. Once you obtain Social Security benefits, you will eventually be eligible for Medicare coverage.

If you have either individual or group disability benefits, you will have to submit much of the same information. If your group benefits are work related, the process will be handled through your employer. You may be required to go on short-term disability before your long-term disability claim begins, and you may be required to use up any sick leave you have accrued. If you go on long-term disability, the insurance carrier may require you to apply for Social Security as well.

Carol's Story

Carol is the school psychologist who was diagnosed with Sjögren's syndrome and lupus. When she began work in 1989, she did not take the disability insurance offered by her school system. Several years later, when she decided to apply for it, she was turned down. By June 1994, she was unable to work at a full-time job, although she did maintain a small private practice in a town near her home. In July 1995, Carol applied for SSDI benefits, and in February of the following year, she received benefits retroactive to December 1994.

Although it is rare to receive disability on the first try, Carol did a number of things that helped her case. Before she applied, she read information about the process on the SSA Web site and obtained printed information from them. Next, she talked with her doctors to make sure that they agreed with her decision. At the time, she had consulted three different doctors on a regular basis, and although she did not have a firm diagnosis (her diagnosis at that time was unspecified autoimmune disease), all three agreed to write supporting letters for her application. Carol asked her doctors to send her copies of the letters and reviewed them before they were sent out. This turned out to be important, because one of her physicians had dictated his letter directly into the service provided by the Social Security Administration for this purpose, and the letter returned from the transcription service with misinformation. Carol was able to have her doctor correct the mistakes before they became part of her application.

She then got copies of all her medical records from all the doctors she had worked with, including those consultants she considered relevant. She included copies of numerous X ray reports and blood tests with her application. Before she completed the application, she spoke with other people who were receiving benefits to find out what had helped them make their cases. On the application itself, she focused on the specific problems that made it impossible for her to work. She experienced chronic and severe fatigue, weakness, flulike feelings, chest pain and shortness of breath, joint and muscle pain, headaches, asthma, stomach and other gastrointestinal problems, reflux, dizziness, blurry vision, dryness of eyes, nose, and mouth, difficulty sleeping, and herniated discs. The self-reporting of her symptoms was backed up by the physician reports, lab reports, and X rays. She listed all the treatments she had received and the medications she had taken.

Carol receives about seven hundred dollars each month. Social Security reviews her status periodically, and she keeps a list of all her medications and doctor's appointments in preparation for these reviews. She has no other source of income. Carol's advice to anyone considering applying for benefits is to be very organized and to be an active participant in the process. She knows it is not always possible to be organized and active when you feel sick, but in her case, the efforts she made paid off.

There is a postscript to this story. Carol's sister, who also has an autoimmune disease, was turned down when she applied for Social

Security benefits. She had not been as systematic as Carol, and did not monitor the reports that her physicians sent to the SSA. Being methodical will not guarantee that your claim will be approved, but it can help you win your case.

Information and Privacy

The issue of who has access to your medical information is of increasing concern to those who worry about privacy. The information that you submit to either a private disability insurer or to the SSA will be seen by many people, and this may include sensitive information provided by your physician. This is why it is a good idea to review the information, as Carol did, before submitting it.

Once a claim is approved and ongoing, the supporting information required may vary. We know of some private insurers who simply require forms to be completed by your primary physician, and we know of others who require copies of the physician's notes after each visit, as well as any laboratory data.

According to a recent article in the *Boston Globe* (Ross 2002), it is becoming increasingly difficult to know who has access to your personal medical files and how that information is used. The article notes that under the terms of the Family Medical Leave Act, firms with over fifty employees are required to provide up to twelve weeks of unpaid but job-protected medical leave annually. When you request a medical leave, how much you must disclose may vary. If you apply for disability insurance, your privacy is likely to be compromised in exchange for your benefits.

Insurance companies have been known to hire private investigators to try to provide evidence that people are not really disabled. The line between surveillance, harassment, and invasion of privacy can be very thin, and the activities of these investigators can be irritating and even frightening. The insurance company may submit your medical information to their experts and may ask you to have an independent medical examination. If this is the case, information that you share with the examiner is not confidential and will be transmitted to the insurance company.

Although both private disability insurers and the SSA have objective criteria for determining disability status, the interpretation of these criteria may be subjective. We know of one person with Sjögren's syndrome whose benefits were terminated because her physician repeatedly used the word "stable" in his notes. What he meant by that word and the insurance company's interpretation were two completely different things. The physician meant that the patient was not getting worse, but never said that she was able to work. The insurance company equated *stable* with cured.

In this case, the woman was allowed a period of time in which to appeal the insurance company's decision. She hired an attorney who specialized in disability law, and her physician provided extensive evidence that supported his definition of "stable." He made an extensive list of things his patient was no longer able to do and provided detailed reasons, backed up by objective evidence, of why she could not return to work. The patient won the appeal and her benefits were restored. She was emotionally and physically exhausted by the process and afterward was no longer stable. She got worse.

If Your Claims Are Denied

We have no idea how often ongoing claims are terminated or how many claims are denied. Insurance companies are there to make money. If your benefits are denied or terminated there are things you can do:

* Let the company know that you intend to mount a vigorous appeal and that you will not passively accept its decision.

* Hire a lawyer who specializes in this area if possible.

* Document everything you send the insurance company. Send any communication via certified mail and attach the cards that indicate the mail has been received to your copy of the communication.

* Keep a record of any conversations with the insurance company. Use direct quotes and always find out the name and title of the person with whom you are speaking.

* Keep your own evidence—copies of medical files and reports—on hand. Ask your physician for these each time you see him or her.

* Have your doctor be specific about what limitations now prevent you from working, such as, "Patient is unable to concentrate for more than an hour or two on some days,

and even less than that on others," or "In the last year, this patient has had five bacterial infections that have prevented her from working at all for a total of more than ninety days," or "This patient cannot look at a computer for more than forty-five minutes because the glare affects her eyes, and cannot use a mouse due to repetitive strain injury."

* Keep a record of all your medications and treatments.

* See your physician every three or four months so that his or her notes are always up-to-date.

* Give your physician a copy of your resume, so that he or she can compare what you have done in the past with what you are able to do now. Annotate the resume with how and why you are unable to perform the tasks you were previously capable of. You may want to provide a resume for the insurance company as well.

* Get letters from friends or colleagues who knew what you used to be able to do and who can provide objective evidence that you are unable to perform these tasks now.

Work is an important part of life and not being able to work can have serious emotional and financial repercussions. Even if you continue to work full time, it doesn't hurt to make contingency plans.

12

Research: Hope
for the Future

In this chapter, we want to give you an idea of some of the new directions scientists are taking in the search for better treatments and, ultimately, a cure. Sjögren's has been poorly understood for a long time, but the base of knowledge that began to emerge in the Sjögren's laboratories at the National Institutes of Health in the 1960s is just now surging forward to reach new heights in the twenty-first century. Our understanding of all autoimmune disease is increasing, and our hope is that one of many emerging concepts will provide the key to unlock the secrets long held by this disease. There *is* hope.

The Promise of Research

The Sjögren's Syndrome Foundation has already brought leaders together to agree on diagnostic criteria for research purposes, and these leaders are well on their way in forging diagnostic criteria for treatment in a clinical setting. The foundation continues to bring scientists together to stimulate research ideas, promote and support research projects, and offer educational programs for clinicians and patients. The Sjögren's Syndrome Clinic at the National Institute of Dental and Craniofacial Research (part of the NIH) leads an international effort to find answers for those of us with Sjögren's. A number of university medical centers also are searching for answers and offering treatment for patients. These centers use specialists from different departments who are knowledgeable about Sjögren's, communicate with each other about the disease and their mutual patients, and coordinate proper treatment among multiple specialists. Some centers have been launched specifically as Sjögren's syndrome clinics, others as autoimmune centers, others as rheumatology or arthritis centers, and still others as women's health centers.

Before new treatments can be developed, scientists need to understand what causes Sjögren's, how organ damage occurs, and what factors are altered in the disorder. We'll take a look at some of the new areas scientists are investigating. For the latest information on the newest drugs, you should refer to the Sjögren's Syndrome Foundation newsletter or Web site, or your own physician.

Information Gathering

The first step in learning more about a disease is gathering information, and, better yet, devising a way for many scientists to share that information. We have had few statistics on Sjögren's syndrome, and there is still a lack of information and disagreement on some very basic issues. These include determining how many people are really affected, demographics of those affected, and what outcomes might be expected for those with specific symptoms and test results. This dearth of knowledge is beginning to change. Tools for gathering and sharing information are improving, and patient advocacy is leading to increased discussions and planning of research strategies.

Registries

A key tool for making progress in research and expanding information is the database, or registry. The National Institute of Dental and Craniofacial Research is providing support to launch the first registry for Sjögren's. International in scope, this registry will serve as a repository for information and biological specimens and be used as a resource for all investigators. This marks the first time such a vast repository of information on Sjögren's will exist and be readily available. Genetics and the ability to interface with existing databases that focus on other autoimmune diseases will be included so we can learn even more. Strict federal guidelines on privacy will be in effect, and no patient identifiers will be used. Elaine Alexander, rheumatologist and researcher, says such a registry "will provide the catalyst for basic research, drug discovery, and development in this important, but often neglected, autoimmune disease" (Alexander 2002).

National Research Plans

The National Institutes of Health in 2003 released the first-ever Autoimmune Diseases Research Plan, a strategic plan to bring researchers from different medical and science specialties together to examine the complete spectrum of autoimmune diseases as one interrelated group. If someone in neurology is discovering something about multiple sclerosis, it might have an impact on other autoimmune diseases with neurological involvement and symptoms. If someone trained in gynecology is investigating the role of hormones during pregnancy in autoimmune diseases, this can have relevance for the eye specialist who is looking at the impact hormones have on dry eyes in autoimmune disease. This approach could greatly accelerate the dissemination of new research findings.

The NIH Autoimmune Diseases Research Plan is a major step forward for those of us with Sjögren's syndrome. Research in four key areas is delineated:

1. *Etiopathogenesis,* a term scientists use combining *etiology* and *pathogenesis,* meaning the origin, cause, and development of disease, and including research in basic science, immunology, and genetics.

2. Epidemiology, the study of statistics about a disease, including how many have it and who is affected.

3. Clinical studies, or research done with patients, including studies on the effects of specific treatments and deciding if treatments are helpful and if benefits are not outweighed by risks.

4. Education, involving dissemination of information and educational opportunities for patients, scientists, health and medical professionals, and the public.

Just think about all we will learn with federal money helping support these many different but critical areas! Money appropriated by Congress not only goes to federal research programs but is distributed in the form of grants to private individuals and medical research centers.

A National Oral Health Plan was launched in 2002 by the U.S. Department of Health and Human Services and the National Institutes of Health. This second plan proposes research for diseases and conditions affecting oral health, including Sjögren's syndrome.

New Insights and Diagnostic Tools

New insights about Sjögren's will lead to development of better diagnostic tools. Our ability to diagnose Sjögren's syndrome needs to become more sophisticated so more people can be diagnosed earlier, more quickly, and with greater accuracy.

One new technique gaining attention is the analysis of saliva. Research centers are finding that saliva might reveal enough information to become a reliable diagnostic tool and replace more invasive procedures, such as the lip biopsy. You might recall that blood samples were needed at first for determining DNA; now, you only need to swab the inside of your cheek to obtain DNA evidence. One day, a doctor will be able to swab the inside of your mouth and look for variations of genes that might be relevant to what's going on in the disease process (Guttmacher 2002).

A new design might be on the horizon for testing autoantibodies. Currently, physicians must test individually for antinuclear antibodies, such as anti-SSA and anti-SSB for Sjögren's and others linked to different autoimmune disorders. Stanford University has developed an antigen microarray test which provides results on a full spectrum of autoimmune diseases in a single test (Robinson et al. 2002).

Etiology Theories

Developing the most effective treatments for any disease involves understanding the disease process and etiology (origin or cause). Let's take a brief look at some of the theories under investigation as a potential cause for inflammation, dysfunction, and destruction in Sjögren's syndrome.

Apoptosis

Cells, when "born," are programmed to die at their specific times. This occurrence, called *apoptosis,* is a normal process. But what happens if certain cells never die, or they die too soon? And what happens if the body cannot get rid of all of these unwanted cells? Many scientists believe this process occurs in Sjögren's. Examining this process can be important to research and provide potential targets for treatment.

Viruses

Many viruses, both common and uncommon, have been investigated and debated for years as possible culprits in Sjögren's. Dr. Patrick Venables has spent a lifetime focusing on viruses and Sjögren's and says, "there is no convincing evidence for any specific virus in the etiology of Sjögren's syndrome" (Venables 2002). However, he also believes that "Sjögren's syndrome is an unusual response to a common virus infection in a genetically susceptible individual."

Other Environmental Triggers

Researchers have examined environmental triggers either proven or believed to cause other autoimmune diseases. These triggers range from bacteria and viruses to chemicals and hormones. Investigators are searching for similar triggers in Sjögren's.

Hormones

Since 90 percent of those with Sjögren's and 75 percent of those with all autoimmune diseases are women, researchers theorize that hormones must play a role. Hormones have an impact on disease activity for women undergoing hormonal changes (pregnancy, birth of a child, cessation of nursing, menopause, and even during periods of lesser change during menstrual periods). Some scientists believe that altering the estrogen metabolism might prove effective.

Investigators are researching the use of hormones for therapy: Dehydroepiandrosterone, commonly called DHEA, is a weak form of androgen. DHEA has undergone clinical trials but has not yet been proven beneficial in Sjögren's. However, research at Schepens Eye Research Institute is encouraging for the use of androgen to treat dry eyes. Schepens senior scientist David Sullivan believes further investigation into the female-male ratio is needed (Sullivan 2002).

Fetal Cells

Cells from pregnancy can remain and circulate for decades throughout a woman's body. In some people, these circulating cells might trigger an autoimmune reaction. This theory could explain why more women than men are prone to autoimmune disease, although it does not appear to explain why some men are affected. However, since cells cross between a fetus and mother, "foreign" cells might also persist in children. Researchers cautiously suggest a link between these cells and autoimmune disease (Guterman 2001).

New Therapies

The last few years have brought breakthroughs in the understanding of autoimmune diseases and in the development of new therapies for Sjögren's. These therapies range from creating innovative immune-modulating agents to new vistas offered by stem cell and genetics research.

The New Secretogogues

Secretegogues are a class of drugs that induce secretions. In Sjögren's, they target specific receptors in the moisture-producing glands and attempt to trigger glands that are no longer functioning and turn them back on so that they are producing moisture once again. The two newest prescription drugs for dry mouth do just that. Salagen and Evoxac target the muscarinic receptors. These receptors are part of the parasympathetic nervous system and stimulate secretions. They are part of a larger group of receptors called G-protein-coupled receptors that might provide opportunities for therapeutic targets in Sjögren's.

Immunomodulation and the New Anti-Inflammatories

Cytokines, proteins involved in communication within and between cells, are among the newest targets for reducing inflammation. These include the tumor necrosis factor, the interleukins, and the interferons. These proteins might act to stimulate and increase inflammation, and some might also be used as therapeutics to reduce inflammation and treat Sjögren's.

Anti-TNF-Alpha Therapy

We discussed this therapy in chapter 3, but we mention it again because this group of drugs marks a recent breakthrough in attacking inflammation. They work by blocking tumor necrosis factor-alpha, or TNF-Alpha, which is involved in many autoimmune disorders, including Sjögren's. Examples are etanercept (Enbrel) and infliximab (Remicade). New drugs are under development, but as with all drugs, you need to weigh your personal medical history along with the benefits and risks.

Anti-TNF-alpha agents have been shown to dramatically decrease fatigue in Sjögren's (Zandbelt et al. 2002), improve anemia in rheumatoid arthritis, and improve eye and skin symptoms in an autoimmune disorder known as Behcet's disease. Infliximab has shown an effect on dryness in Sjögren's in one uncontrolled trial (Steinfeld 2001).

Interleukins

Many interleukins are under investigation in relation to Sjögren's. For example, Interleukin-10, or IL-10, is a known promoter of cytokine inflammation and creates yet another potential target for exploration in new therapies. Concentrations of Interleukin-2 (IL-2) and Interleukin-6 (IL-6) are significantly higher in Sjögren's syndrome patients and are associated with inflammation and destruction of salivary glands. Researchers have found that administering interferon reduces both IL-2 and IL-6 in Sjögren's (Streckfus et al. 2001).

Interferon

Trials were recently launched for use of interferon-alpha lozenges to stimulate saliva. Researchers are finding improvement in salivary flow, and investigations continue into this possible treatment.

Developing Antibodies for Specific Targets

Monoclonal antibodies might have a role in treating disease. These are proteins produced through recombinant technologies that have high specificity for a selected target. For example, rituximab targets CD20 antibodies and is effective in non-Hodgkin's lymphoma. Infliximab (Remicade), which acts against TNF-alpha, is also a monoclonal antibody. Following recent successes, scientists will surely devise other antibodies to treat Sjögren's.

Vaccines

The National Cancer Institute at the National Institutes of Health is testing a vaccine for B-cell lymphomas. This vaccine does not prevent cancer from developing (like other vaccines that prevent illness), but it is designed to strengthen the body's attack on a cancer that has already developed. Early results indicate success of the vaccine, but testing is incomplete.

Stem Cells

The use of stem cells to treat and cure disease is one of the newest and most exciting frontiers in medicine. Stem cells have been proven to help treat severe autoimmune diseases and have tremendous potential for treating and curing many diseases.

Stem cells are undefined cells that may differentiate to form any type of cell in the body. Human pluripotent stem cell research could have enormous repercussions some day. If you have an immune system whose cells are not functioning correctly, organs that are dysfunctional, or tissue that has been destroyed, new cells and tissue could be generated using stem cells. In addition, human pluripotent stem cell research could lead to a better understanding of cell processes. New therapies could be developed more easily, as potential medications are first tested on human cell lines before being tried in animals and humans. The possibilities are many, and the potential impact tremendous.

Right now, transplanting stem cells into people is a difficult and high-risk procedure. It has proven successful in some cases and shows promise, but much more work needs to be done. This area of medicine has become controversial in the United States, because some people are opposed on ethical grounds, automatically equating the gathering of stem cells with increased abortion. Stem cells can come from many sources, including the placenta of a baby (which would usually just be thrown away), embryos and fetal tissue (which might be produced from failed fertilization attempts), and even from adults. Adult stem cells, however, have not yet proven to show as great a potential for research and therapies.

Genetics Theory

We've already taken a look at genes that might influence development of Sjögren's syndrome and other autoimmune diseases. Researchers are looking into the possibility that a correlation between Sjögren's and specific genes might be found. Genetic mutations might also have an impact, and these mutations could involve any number of processes that are linked with Sjögren's syndrome.

Finally, success in learning how to decipher the entire human genetic system, or the human genome, will provide us even more information about Sjögren's. Traditional genetics has looked at genes that are directly responsible for disease; the scope of the human genome, however, is much broader and will allow scientists to examine the entire picture of your genetic makeup. As an example of the vast difference in approaches, we might compare the process of having looked at only one star or one planet versus being able to see the whole solar system, which provides a very different perspective and tells a different story. For complex diseases such as Sjögren's syndrome, the impact of this new expanding field of science could be profound.

The Human Genome

Deciphering the human genome will revolutionize medicine. In the year 2000, scientists announced that they could read the human genetic map. Genes are the basic units of heredity, and your genome is your genetic map. This map is found in every living cell, and now every part of this map can be identified.

The Human Genome Project is the international effort by scientists to map and sequence all human genes. The map is complete, and scientists believe completion of gene sequencing will be accomplished in 2003. Eventually, it will be possible to identify genes and their proteins that are associated with a specific disease by comparing the genes of patients with a "standard" sequence from healthy individuals. The Human Genome Project will not only provide a diagnostic tool to find out who might be susceptible to certain diseases; more than that, it will allow doctors and scientists to take medicine a step further and look into novel and effective treatments for those same diseases.

What could this mean for the approximately four million Americans who suffer from Sjögren's syndrome? There are no clear answers, but this accomplishment opens a major window for possibilities and hope that never existed before for anyone who suffers from any disease, including Sjögren's syndrome. Bruce Baum, chief of the Gene Therapy and Therapeutics Branch at NIDCR, the National Institutes of Health, says, "The genome project will allow an explosion in a bunch of fields related to the management of Sjögren's syndrome, ranging from immunology to cell biology" (Baum 2000).

Now that we can study all genes in existence, scientists' understanding of the influence of genes on Sjögren's and how genes might be manipulated to help those with autoimmune diseases will open up new realms of possibility for treatment. Dr. Stuart Kassan of the University of Colorado Health Sciences Center in Denver and chair of the Sjögren's Syndrome Foundation's Medical and Scientific Advisory Board says the Human Genome Project will stimulate research into autoimmunity and allow us to better correlate symptoms and outcome. Kassan says this new knowledge will encourage the burgeoning of drug development and progress in genetic engineering, through which a person's genetic makeup might eventually be changed to actually block autoimmune disease (Kassan 2000).

Gene Therapy

Gene therapy can be used to treat, cure, or prevent disorders that are genetically related. In Sjögren's syndrome, research into gene therapy is focusing on making salivary glands function correctly. Gene therapy involves the transfer of genetic material; for example, inserting proteins such as cytokines into salivary glands to change the way the glands function. The difficulty for researchers right now is the manner in which those genes are transferred. Once a means for transferring those genes without causing patient reactions is found, and scientists learn to control how those genes express themselves and function, saliva production could improve. Baum believes that with the many bright people dedicated to grappling with these questions, we'll find a way to make this therapy work for Sjögren's patients. He hopes to be overseeing clinical trials for gene transfer in people with Sjögren's in the next decade (Baum 2000).

Artificial Glands

Development of artificial glands is a future possibility. Bladders in dogs have been successfully replaced with artificial bladders, and bladders are complicated organs. Baum believes there is future promise in creating new, functional glands in Sjögren's (Baum 2000).

Complementary Therapies

Complementary therapies are increasingly gaining acceptance and becoming a focal point for scientific investigation. A new institute at the National Institutes of Health was created in recognition of the growing acceptance of complementary therapies and to test such therapies on diseases, such as Sjögren's syndrome. The National Center for Complementary and Alternative Medicine addresses practices and theories that are outside the realm of conventional medicine and tries to answer key questions about the benefits of using herbs, vitamins, electromagnetic fields, mind-body connections, and energy therapies.

Research Support

Research is carried out using both private and public funds. Foundations such as the Sjögren's Syndrome Foundation raise and collect funds for research; scientists, clinicians, fellows, and students can apply for grants which are reviewed by the foundation's Medical and Scientific Advisory Board and awarded on a regular basis. University and other research centers often use a mixture of private donations and state and federal funding. The National Institutes of Health, which is funded by Congress, supports the majority of health research in the United States.

If you're reading this book, you already want to help yourself and perhaps others in your family, circle of friends, or those at large who have Sjögren's syndrome. If you have Sjögren's syndrome, you can help by participating in clinical trials. You don't have to have Sjögren's to help by volunteering or donating dollars to organizations that support research.

Participating in Clinical Studies

Clinical trials are studies evaluating the benefits of treatments on human beings, an important step before deciding if a treatment will work and if the benefits outweigh the risks. Clinical trials are required before a drug or other treatment can be marketed and sold. These trials are very carefully regulated by federal guidelines.

If it weren't for clinical trials, those who suffer from diseases such as Sjögren's syndrome would have little hope of potential treatments and an eventual cure. "At present, we have no truly effective treatment, and the prospects for new modalities depend entirely on clinical trials," says Dr. Michael Lemp, a Counselor for the Sjögren's Syndrome Foundation's Medical and Scientific Advisory Board (Lemp 2000).

The National Library of Medicine has launched a clinical trials database so that information on clinical trials can be easily obtained by patients, physicians, and scientists. This database includes both federally and privately funded trials. It will prove particularly beneficial for research into Sjögren's, in which better devices for sharing knowledge about potential treatments and research is critical.

If you are considering participation in a clinical trial, it's important to be an educated consumer. Understand the design and purpose of the trial, the criteria for participation, and most of all, the risks involved. You should always talk to your doctor beforehand, to examine your personal medical history in relation to potential risks.

Volunteering

Every one of us has something we can do to contribute to making life better for those with Sjögren's syndrome. You can distribute materials to local health care workers and physicians, contact local media for publicity about Sjögren's, write letters to Congress supporting initiatives that will help those with Sjögren's, or provide your name and contact information to a foundation as a resource for support or information. Organizations such as the Sjögren's Syndrome

Foundation, the American Autoimmune Related Diseases Association, and other groups serving related disorders can let you know specific ways in which you can help.

Financial Support

Donating money to research centers and foundations helps those organizations to function and continue the research that is so critical to future progress.

A Final Word

We hope we've given you a glimpse of the vast array of fresh and new ideas that researchers are debating and investigating. Not all of these ideas will pan out. Some may die a quiet death soon after the publication of this book, and we have probably over-looked some ideas that may prove to be important, but many will come to fruition or at least will provide the basis for other treatments that do. Philip C. Fox, oral health specialist and researcher, says that for Sjögren's patients, "New and future therapies will be directed at the underlying cause and mechanisms of the disorder, rather than at the symptoms. Obviously, once we know the cause and understand the mechanisms, this will make the job much easier! We are getting a better understanding of the disease process and this translates into becoming testable" (Fox 2000). This is wonderful news for those of us who have had treatments only for the symptoms of Sjögren's.

New doors to new information and possibilities are opening all the time, providing greater hope for the future than ever before. The breakthroughs of today and those on the horizon bring the message of future promise to those of us with Sjögren's syndrome. Living with Sjögren's syndrome will, indeed, become better, and a cure will be found.

Resources

Resources include nonprofit foundations, treatment centers, the Internet, support groups, and your library or bookstore. Always check with your doctor about medical advice, and don't forget that one of the best resources could be your own doctor and the nurses and other health care professionals you will meet.

Consider the Source

As you examine resources, always consider the source. Is the source knowledgeable? What is the individual's or sponsoring group's affiliation? Area of expertise? Credentials? Training? Purpose? Is the group trying to sell something, or does it have another bias that might affect the information provided? Is the information up-to-date? Nonprofits focusing on disease should have medical boards to authorize and review information.

We cannot list all sources, so we will provide only a few favorites to get you started. Remember, Internet addresses can change frequently, and new Web sites appear and disappear quickly. We encourage you to contact the Sjögren's Syndrome Foundation and other associations listed to learn about additional excellent sources of information. These associations have regular publications and Web sites that list currently available and new sources.

The Sjögren's Syndrome Foundation (SSF), the first listing in this section, offers contacts and support groups around the United States and in cities around the world. Some contacts specialize in specific topics of interest to Sjögren's patients. SSF's Web site can lead you to international Sjögren's syndrome organizations and groups. SSF also offers regional and national symposia, which provide an opportunity not only to learn more about Sjögren's but to meet experts and other patients.

Foundations for Sjögren's Syndrome

Sjögren's Syndrome Foundation
8120 Woodmont Avenue, Suite 530
Bethesda, MD 20814
Phone: (301) 718-0300 or (800) 475-6473
Web site: www.sjogrens.org

American Autoimmune Related Diseases Association
22100 Gratiot Avenue
East Detroit, MI 48021
Phone: (586) 776-3900
Web site: www.aarda.org

Arthritis Foundation
1330 West Peachtree Street
Atlanta, GA 30309
Phone: (800) 283-7800
Web site: www.arthritis.org

National Institutes of Health

NIH Sjögren's Syndrome Clinic
National Institute of Dental and Craniofacial Research
10 Center Drive, MSC 1190
Building 10, Room 1N113
Bethesda, MD 20892-1190
Phone: (301) 435-8528

Web site:
wwwdir.nidcr.nih.gov/dirweb/gttb/sjogrens/Sjogrenindex.asp

National Institute of Dental and Craniofacial Research
NIH, 45 Center Drive, MSC 6400
Building 45, Room 4AS-25
Bethesda, MD 20892-6400
Phone: (301) 496-4261
Web site: www.nidcr.nih.gov

National Eye Institute
NIH, 2020 Vision Place
Bethesda, MD 20892-3655
Phone: (301) 496-5248
Web site: www.nei.nih.gov

National Institute of Allergy and Infectious Diseases
NIH, 31 Center Drive, MSC 2520
Building 31, Room 7A-50
Bethesda, MD 20892-2520
Phone: (301) 496-5717
Web site: www.niaid.nih.gov

National Institute of Arthritis and Musculoskeletal and Skin Diseases
Information Clearinghouse
NIH, 1 AMS Circle
Bethesda, MD 20892-3675
Phone: (301) 495-4484 or (877) 226-4267
Web site: www.nih.gov/niams

National Institute of Neurological Disorders and Stroke
NIH, Office of Communications and Public Liaison
PO Box 5801
Bethesda, MD 20824
Phone: (800) 352-9424
Web site: www.ninds.nih.gov

Office of Research on Women's Health
9000 Rockville Pike
Building 1, Room 201
Bethesda, MD 20892

Phone: (301) 402-1770
Web site: www4.od.nih.gov/orwh/

National Center for Complementary and Alternative Medicine
NCCAM Clearinghouse
PO Box 7923
Gaithersburg, MD 20898
Phone: (888) 644-6226
Web site: http://nccam.nih.gov

National Human Genome Research Institute
9000 Rockville Pike
Building 31, Room 4B09
31 Center Drive, MSC 2152
Bethesda, MD 20892-2152
Phone: (301) 402-0911
Web site: www.genome.gov

National Cancer Institute
Public Inquiries Office, Suite 3036A
6116 Executive Boulevard, MSC8322
Bethesda, MD 20892-8322
Phone: (800) 422-6237
Web site: www.nci.nih.gov

Medical and Other Information

Social Security Administration
Web site: www.ssa.gov

NIH Clinical Center
Phone: (800) 411-1222
Web site: http://clinicalstudies.info.nih.gov

National Oral Health Information Clearinghouse
Phone: (301) 402-7364
Web site: www.nohic.nidcr.nih.gov

National Health Information Center
Phone: (301) 565-4167 or (800) 336-4797
Web site: www.healthfinder.gov

Combined Health Information Database
Web site: www.chid.nih.gov

National Library of Medicine, NIH
Web site: www.nlm.nih.gov/
Web site listing clinical trials within and outside the federal government
www.clinical/trials.gov

The National Women's Health Information Center
The Office on Women's Health
US Department of Health and Human Services
Phone: (800) 994-9662
Web site: www.4women.gov

Intelihealth
Web site: www.intelihealth.com

Mayo Clinic
Web site: www.mayoclinic.com

Johns Hopkins University Autoimmune Disease Research Center
Web site: http://autoimmune.pathology.jhmi.edu

WebMD and Medscape
Web site: www.webmd.com
www.medscape.com

MedicineNet
Web site: www.medicinenet.com

Lab Tests Online
Web site: http://labtestsonline.org/index.html

Centerwatch
Web site: www.centerwatch.com

Dry-Dot-Org
Web site: www.dry.org

Internet Listservs

Two e-mail listservs provide support and information for those with Sjögren's syndrome and their friends and family members. Information on both lists and how to join is available at www.dry.org.

SS-L is an e-mail list focusing on medical information. It's moderated and has over 700 subscribers.

TalkSjo is a support list that provides more conversation and sociability online and was set up to help those with Sjögren's feel less isolated.

Related Disorders

Lupus Foundation of America
1300 Pickard Drive, Suite 200
Rockville, MD 20850
Phone: (301) 670-9292 or (800) 558-0121
Web site: www.lupus.org

Scleroderma Foundation
12 Kent Way, Suite 101
Byfield, MA 01922
Phone: (978) 463-5843 or (800) 722-4673
Web site: www.scleroderma.org

Scleroderma Research Foundation
2320 Bath Street, Suite 315
Santa Barbara, CA 93105
Phone: (805) 563-2402
Web site: www.srfcure.org

The Thyroid Society
7515 South Main Street, Suite 545
Houston, TX 77030
Phone: (713) 799-9909 or (800) 849-7643
Website: http://the-thyroid-society.org

Thyroid Foundation of America
Ruth Sleeper Hall, RSL 350
40 Parkman Street
Boston, MA 02114

Phone: (617) 726-8500 or (800) 832-8321
Web site: www.allthyroid.org

The National Multiple Sclerosis Society
733 Third Avenue
New York, NY 10017
Phone: (800) 344-4867
Web site: www.nationalmssociety.org

The Neuropathy Association
60 E. 42nd Street, Suite 942
New York, NY 10165
Phone: (212) 962-0662 or (800) 247-6968
Web site: www.neuropathy.org

Crohn's and Colitis Foundation of America
386 Park Avenue South, 17th Floor
New York, NY 10016-8804
Phone: (212) 685-3440 or (800) 932-2423
Web site: www.ccfa.org

American Liver Foundation
75 Maiden Lane, Suite 603
New York, NY 10038
Phone: (973) 256-2550 or (800) 443-7222
Webs ite: www.liverfoundation.org

Myositis Association of America
1233 20th St. NW, Suite 402
Washington, DC 20036
Phone: (202) 887-0082
Web site: www.myositis.org

The American Fibromyalgia Syndrome Association
6380 E. Tanque Verde, Suite D
Tucson, AZ 85715
Phone: (520) 733-1570
Web site: www.afsafund.org

The National Fibromyalgia Association
2238 N. Glassell Street, Suite D
Orange, CA 92865

Phone: (714) 921-0150
Web site: http://fmaware.org

The American Association for Chronic Fatigue Syndrome
515 Minor Avenue, Suite 18
Seattle, WA 98104
Phone: (206) 781-3544
Web site: www.aacfs.org

The TMJ Association
PO Box 26770
Milwaukee, WI 53226
Web site: www.tmj.org

Lymphoma Research Foundation
8800 Venice Boulevard, Suite 207
Los Angeles, CA 90034
Phone: (310) 204-7040 or (800) 500-9976
Web site: www.lymphoma.org

The Leukemia & Lymphoma Society
1311 Mamaroneck Avenue
White Plains, NY 10605
Phone: (914) 949-5213
Web site: www.leukemia-lymphoma.org

Treatment Centers

Duke University Sjögren's Syndrome Clinic
Duke University Medical Center,
Rheumatology, Allergy, and Clinical Immunology
Durham, NC
Phone: (919) 684-4499
Web site: http://rheumatology.duke.edu/home.asp?dividionID=54

Hospital for Joint Diseases, Rheumatology
New York, NY
Phone: (212) 598-6000
Web site:
www.msnyuhealth.org/hospitals/hjd/html/sjogrens_syndrome.html

Johns Hopkins University Autoimmune Disease Research Center
Baltimore, MD
Web site: http://autoimmune.pathology.jhmi.edu

Lowenstein Foundation Sjögren's Center
Mount Sinai Medical Center, Division of Rheumatology
New York, NY
Phone: (212) 241-3173
Web site: www.mssm.edu/medicine/rheumatology/patients/shtml

NIH Sjögren's Syndrome Clinic
National Institute of Dental and Craniofacial Research
Bethesda, MD
Phone: (301) 435-8528
Web site:
wwwdir.nidcr.nih.gov/dirweb/gttb/sjogrens/Sjogrenindex.asp

Sjögren's Multi-Specialty Referral Center
Baylor College of Dentistry
Baylor University Medical Center
Dallas, TX
Phone: (214) 828-8490
Web site: www.tambed.edu/sjogrens.htm

The Cleveland Clinic Foundation
Department of Rheumatic and Immunologic Diseases
Cleveland, OH
Phone: (216) 444-2200 or (800) 223-2273, ext. 48950
Web site: www.clevelandclinic.org/arthritis/default.htm

University of Connecticut
Division of Rheumatology
Farmington, CT
Phone: (860) 523-7344
Web site: www2.uchc.edu/%7Erheum/info.html

University of Florida Center for Autoimmune Diseases
Gainesville, FL
Phone: (352) 392-4681

University of Pennsylvania Sjögren's Syndrom Clinic
Presbyterian Medical Center
University of Pennsylvania Health System
Philadelphia, PA
Phone: (215) 662-8000
Web site: www.uphs.upenn.edu

Dry Mouth Clinics

Salivary Dysfunction Clinic
Baylor College of Dentistry
Dallas, TX
Phone: (214) 828-8490
Web site: www.tambed.edu/salivary

Salivary Dysfunction Center
University of Rochester Medical Center
Rochester, NY
Phone: (716) 275-7978
Web site:
www.urmc.rochester.edu/Dentistry/EDD/training/saldys.html

Xerostomia Clinic
University of Minnesota, School of Dentistry
Department of Oral Medicine
Minneapolis, MN
Phone: (612) 625-0693
Web site:
www.dentistry.umn.edu/community/Xerostomia_Clinic445.html

Dry Eye Clinics

Casey Eye Institute
Portland, OR
Phone: (503) 494-5023
Web site: www.ohsuhealth.com/cei/research/inflammatory.asp

Dry Eye and Tear Research Center
St. Paul-Ramsey Medical Center
St. Paul, MN
Phone: (651) 254-3036

Schepens Eye Research Institute
Harvard Medical School
Boston, MA
Phone: (617) 912-0100
Web site: www.eri.harvard.edu

Publications

The New Sjögren's Syndrome Handbook, edited by Steven Carsons and Elaine K. Harris, produced by the Sjögren's Syndrome Foundation and published by Oxford University Press, 1998.

A Delicate Balance: Living Successfully with Chronic Illness, by Susan Milstrey Wells, Perseus Publishing, first published 1998.

Understanding Sjögren's Syndrome, by Sue Dauphin, Pixel Press, 1993.

Sick and Tired of Feeling Sick and Tired: Living with Invisible Chronic Illness, by Paul J. Donogue and Mary E. Siegel, W. W. Norton and Company, 1992.

You Are Not Your Illness: Seven Principles for Meeting the Challenge, by Linda Noble Topf, Hal Zina Bennett, and Bernie S. Siegel, published by Fireside, 1995.

We Are Not Alone: Learning to Live with Chronic Illness, by Sefra K. Pitzele, Workman Publishing, first published 1985.

References

Alexander, E. 1998. Neurologic disease in Sjögren's syndrome. In *The Handbook of Clinical Neurology: Systemic Diseases*. Edited by M. J. Aminoff and C. G. Goetz. New York: Elsevier Science Publishing.

———. 2002. Personal communication, 4 May.

Ahmed S., B. Hissong, D. Verthelyi, K. Donner, K. Becker, and E. Karpuzoglu-Sahin. 1999. Gender and risk of autoimmune diseases: Possible role of estrogenic compounds. *Environmental Health Perspectives* 7:681–686.

American Psychiatric Association (APA). 2000. *Diagnostic and Statistical Manual of Mental Disorders*. 4th ed. Text revision. Washington: American Psychiatric Association.

Baum, B. 2000. Personal communication, July.

Benson, H. 1996. *Timeless Healing*. New York: Fireside Books.

Berman, R. 2001. Personal communication, November.

Boston Healthcare Associates. 1996. Survey in cooperation with the Sjögren's Syndrome Foundation, printed by Boston Healthcare Associates.

Buyon, J. 1998. Pregnancy in women with Sjögren's syndrome: Neonatal problems. In *The New Sjögren's Syndrome Handbook*, edited by S. Carsons and E. Harris. New York: Oxford University Press.

Carsons, S., and E. Harris, eds. 1998. *The New Sjögren's Syndrome Handbook*. New York: Oxford University Press.

Cassileth, B., E. Lusk, D. Miller, L. Brown, and C. Miller. 1985. Psychosocial correlates of survival in advanced malignant disease. *New England Journal of Medicine* 312:1551–1555.

Cousins, N. 1979. *Anatomy of an Illness*. New York: Bantam Books.

Domar, A., and H. Dreher. 1996. *Healing Mind, Healthy Woman*. New York: Delta Books.

Dubovsky, S. 1981. In *Understanding Behavior in Health and Illness*, edited by R. Simons and H. Pardes. 2nd ed. Baltimore: Williams and Wilkins.

Eskrels, D. 1998. Disorders of the gastrointestinal system. In *The New Sjögren's Syndrome Handbook*, edited by S. Carsons and E. Harris. Oxford: Oxford University Press.

Fox, P. 2000. Personal communication, July.

Fox, R., ed. 1992. *Rheumatic Disease Clinics of North America, Sjögren's Syndrome* 18, 3. Philadelphia: Saunders Company, Harcourt Brace Jovanovich.

Gaylin, W. 1979. *Feelings*. New York: Ballantine Books.

———. 1984. *The Rage Within: Anger in Modern Life*. New York: Simon and Schuster.

Goodman, E., and P. O'Brien. 2000. *I Know Just What You Mean*. New York: Simon and Schuster.

Greene, W. 1966. The psychosocial setting of the development of leukemia and lymphoma. *Annals of the New York Academy of Science* 125:794–801.

Greene, W., L. Young, and S. Swisher. 1956. Psychological factors and reticuloendothelial disease: Observations on a group of men with lymphomas and leukemia. *Psychosomatic Medicine* 18:284–303.

Guterman, L. 2001. A generational battle: Cells from her children may harm a mother years later. *Chronicle of Higher Education* 6 April 2001; 47:A21–A22.

Guttmacher, A. 2002. Presentation before NIH NIAMS Coalition.

Haarala, M., A. Alanen, M. Hietarinta, and P. Kiiholma. 2000. Lower urinary tract symptoms in patients with Sjögren's syndrome and systemic lupus erythematosus. *International Urogynecology Journal and Pelvic Floor Dysfunction* 11:84–86.

Hafen, B., K. Karren, K. Frandsen, and N. Smith. 1996. *Mind/Body Health*. Boston: Allen and Bacon.

Hahn, B. 2000. On the edge of the millennium: Prospects and problems for our patients and us. *Arthritis and Rheumatism* 43(4):715–719.

Hansen, L., U. Prakash, T. Colby. 1989. Pulmonary lymphoma in Sjögren's syndroms. *Mayo Clin Proc* 1898 Aug; 64(8):920–31.

Hess, E. 1999. Are there environmental forms of systemic auto-immune diseases? *Environmental Health Perspectives* 7:709–712.

Holladay, S. 1999. Prenatal immunotoxicant exposure and postnatal autoimmune disease. *Environmental Health Perspectives* 7:687–692.

Horstman, J. 1999. *The Arthritis Foundation's Guide to Alternative Therapies*. Atlanta: The Arthritis Foundation.

Jonsson, R., H. Haga, and T. Gordon. 2001. Sjögren's syndrome. In *Arthritis and Allied Conditions*. 14th ed. Edited by W. J. Koopman. Philadelphia and New York: Lippincott, Williams and Wilkins.

Kabat-Zinn, J. 1990. *Full Catastrophe Living*. New York: Delta Books.

Kalk, W., A. Vissink, B. Stegenga, H. Bootsma, A. Nieuw Amerongen, and C. Kallenberg. 2001. Sialometry and sialochemistry: Diagnostic tools for Sjögren's syndrome. *Annals of the Rheumatic Diseases* 60(12):1110–1116.

Kassan, S. 2000. Personal communication, July.

Kleinman, A. 1988. *The Illness Narratives*. New York: Basic Books.

Kushner, H. 1981. *When Bad Things Happen to Good People.* New York: Avon Books.

Lazare, A. 1987. Shame and humiliation in the medical encounter. *Archives of Internal Medicine* 147(9):1653–1658.

Lemp, M. 1999. Personal correspondence, 27 September.

———. 2000. Personal communication, 3 February.

Lerner, H. 1997. *The Dance of Anger.* New York: Harper Perennial.

Lown, B. 1996. *The Lost Art of Healing.* Boston: Houghton Mifflin Company.

Mazer, H. 2001. Personal communication, May.

Medical Economics Company. 2001. *Physicians' Desk Reference.* 55th ed. Montvale, N.J.: Medical Economics Company.

Meisler, J. 2001. Toward optimal health: The experts discuss dry eye syndrome; an interview with M. Dana, D. Sullivan, and A. Parke. *Journal of Women's Health and Gender-Based Medicine* 10:8.

Mohan N., E. Edwards, T. Cupps, P. Oliverio, G. Sandberg, H. Crayton, J. Richert, and J. Siegel. 2001. Demyelination occurring during anti-tumor necrosis factor alpha therapy for inflammatory arthritides. *Arthritis and Rheumatism* 44(12):2862–2869.

Nathanson, R. 2002. Personal communication, January.

Ornstein, R., and D. Sobel. 1989. *Healthy Pleasures.* Reading, Mass.: Perseus Books.

Parks, C., K. Conrad, and G. Cooper. 1999. Occupational exposure to crystalline silica and autoimmune disease. *Environmental Health Perspectives* 7:793–802.

Phillips, R. 2001. *Coping with Lupus.* New York: Avery Books.

Piburn, G. 1999. *Beyond Chaos: One Man's Journey Alongside His Chronically Ill Wife.* Atlanta: Arthritis Foundation.

Pillemer, S. 2002. Personal communication, September.

Politi, Z. 2000. Hearing loss in Sjögren's syndrome patients: A comparative study. *Clinical and Experimental Rheumatology* 18:725–728.

Robinson W., C. Digennaro, W. Hueber, B. Haab, M. Kamachi, E. Dean, S. Fournel, D. Fong, M. Genovese, H. DeVegvar, K.

Skriner, D. Hirschberg, R. Morris, S. Muller, G. Pruijn, W. Van Venrooij, J. Smolen, P. Brown, L. Steinman, and P. Utz. 2002. Autoantigen microarrays for multiplex characterization of autoantibody response. *Nature Medicine* 8:295–301.

Ross, S. 2002. Medical files not always safe at work. *Boston Globe,* 26 May, G1.

Rumpf, T. 1997. *Moisture Seekers Newsletter*, September, 5.

Schaumberg, D., J. Buring, D. Sullivan, and M. Dana. 2001. Hormone Replacement Therapy and Dry Eye Syndrome. *Journal of the American Medical Association* 286:2114–9.

Selye, H. 1974. *Stress without Distress*. Philadelphia and New York: J. B. Lippincott Company.

Sieder, J. 2000. The Disability Dance. *Arthritis Today,* July-August, 153–158.

Skevington, S. 1995. *Psychology of Pain*. Chichester, England: John Wiley and Sons.

Sontag, S. 1977. *Illness As Metaphor*. New York: Farrar, Straus and Giroux.

Spijkervet, F., W. Kalk, A. Vissink, H. Bootsma, C. Kallenberg, and J. Roodenburg. 2002. Diagnostic value of parotid gland sialography in Sjögren's syndrome, Department of Oral and Maxillofacial Surgery and Internal Medicine, University Hospital Groningen, the Netherlands. Poster presented at VIIIth International Symposium on Sjögren's Syndrome, Kanazawa, Japan.

Steinfeld, S., P. Demols, I. Salmon, R. Kiss, and T. Appelboom. 2001. Infliximab in patients with primary Sjögren's syndrome: A pilot study. *Arthritis and Rheumatism* 44:2371–2375.

Sternberg, E. 2001. *The Balance Within*. New York: W. H. Freeman and Company.

Streckfus, C., L. Bigler, M. Navazesh, and I. Al-Hashimi. 2001. Cytokine concentrations in stimulated whole saliva among patients with primary Sjögren's syndrome, secondary Sjögren's syndrome, and patients with primary Sjögren's syndrome receiving varying doses of interferon for symptomatic treatment of the condition: A preliminary study. *Clinical Oral Investigations* 5:133–135.

Sullivan, D. 2002. Personal communication, 16 May.

Szasz, S. 1991. *Living with It: Why You Don't Have to Be Healthy to Be Happy.* Buffalo, New York: Prometheus Books.

Takagi, H., M. Ochoa, L. Zhou, T. Helfman, H. Murata, and V. Falanga. 1995. Enhanced collagen synthesis and transcription by peak E, a contaminant of L-tryptophan preparations associated with the eosinophilia myalgia syndrome epidemic. *Journal of Clinical Investigation* 96:2120–2125.

Talal, N. 1998. *Lymphoma in Sjögren's Syndrome Handbook,* edited by S. Carsons and E. Harris. New York: Oxford University Press. 105–7.

Tompkins, F. 2002. Personal communication, January.

Venables, P. 2002. Viruses and Sjögren's syndrome. Paper presented at the VIIIth International Symposium on Sjögren's Syndrome, Kanazawa, Japan.

Vitali C., S. Bombardieri, R. Jonsson, H. Moutsopoulos, E. Alexander, S. Carson, T. Daniels, P. Fox, R. Fox, S. Kassan, S. Pillemer, N. Talal, and M. Weisman. 2002. Classification criteria for Sjögren's syndrome: A revised version of the European criteria proposed by the American-European Consensus Group. *Annals of the Rheumatic Diseases* 61(6):554–558.

Wallace, D. 1995. *The Lupus Book: A Guide for Patients and Their Families.* Oxford: Oxford University Press.

Wells, S. 2000. *A Delicate Balance: Living Successfully with Chronic Illness.* Cambridge, Mass.: Perseus Books.

Wilson, J. 2001. Personal communication, February.

Winter, W. 1995. Gland alert. *Diabetes Forecast* 48:34–39.

Zandbelt, M., P. deWilde, C. Hoyng, P. Van Damme, L. Van de Putte, and F. van den Hoogen. 2002. Etanercept (Enbrel) treatment in primary Sjögren's syndrome: Preliminary results of an open label pilot study. Poster presented at the VIIIth International Symposium on Sjögren's Syndrome, Kanazawa, Japan.

Index

Teri P. Rumpf, Ph.D., is a clinical psychologist and writer who has done research and authored numerous articles and essays on the psychological aspects of illness. Formerly on the faculty of the University of Massachusetts Medical Center and in private practice, she was interested in how illness affects life long before she heard of Sjögren's syndrome or knew she would have it.

Katherine Morland Hammitt, MA, a journalist and Past President of the Sjögren's Syndrome Foundation, currently serves as its public policy director. She is also a member of the coordinating committee for research in autoimmune diseases for the National Institutes of Health and helped author its strategic research plan. Her interest in and advocacy for Sjögren's syndrome spring from her own experience with the illness. She has devoted nearly twenty years to improving diagnosis and treatment and finding a cure for all those who suffer from this serious disease.

Some Other
New Harbinger Titles

Stop Worrying Abour Your Health, Item SWYH $14.95

The Vulvodynia Survival Guide, Item VSG $15.95

The Multifidus Back Pain Solution, Item MBPS $12.95

Move Your Body, Tone Your Mood, Item MBTM $17.95

The Chronic Illness Workbook, Item CNIW $16.95

Coping with Crohn's Disease, Item CPCD $15.95

The Woman's Book of Sleep, Item WBS $14.95

The Trigger Point Therapy Workbook, Item TPTW $19.95

Fibromyalgia and Chronic Myofascial Pain Syndrome, second edition, Item FMS2 $19.95

Kill the Craving, Item KC $18.95

Rosacea, Item ROSA $13.95

Thinking Pregnant, Item TKPG $13.95

Shy Bladder Syndrome, Item SBDS $13.95

Help for Hairpullers, Item HFHP $13.95

Coping with Chronic Fatigue Syndrome, Item CFS $13.95

The Stop Smoking Workbook, Item SMOK $17.95

Multiple Chemical Sensitivity, Item MCS $16.95

Breaking the Bonds of Irritable Bowel Syndrome, Item IBS $14.95

Parkinson's Disease and the Art of Moving, Item PARK $16.95

The Addiction Workbook, Item AWB $18.95

The Interstitial Cystitis Survival Guide, Item ICS $15.95

Illness and the Art of Creative Self-Expression, Item EXPR $13.95

Don't Leave it to Chance, Item GMBL $13.95

Call **toll free, 1-800-748-6273,** or log on to our online bookstore at **www.newharbinger.com** to order. Have your Visa or Mastercard number ready. Or send a check for the titles you want to New Harbinger Publications, Inc., 5674 Shattuck Ave., Oakland, CA 94609. Include $4.50 for the first book and 75¢ for each additional book, to cover shipping and handling. (California residents please include appropriate sales tax.) Allow two to five weeks for delivery.

Prices subject to change without notice.